AF844087

Praise for *The Naked Eye*

"I found *The Naked Eye* really helpful in deciding whether to undergo laser eye surgery."

"I love how the book is written in conversational layperson's language and it makes you feel as though you are just having a chat with someone who has a lot of knowledge in the area."

"This is an easy to read, enjoyable book for anyone interested in the evolution of eye surgery as well as for people seriously evaluating laser surgery."

"This is a very informative book that will debunk any preconceived ideas and concerns that the reader may have about eye laser surgery."

"This excellent read will give any reader a sound understanding of contemporary surgical correction of vision, its history, its heroes and a glimpse into its future."
Clinical and Experimental Optometry

"This book admirably serves its purpose to educate prospective patients, as well as medical practitioners in ophthalmology and optometry, regarding laser vision correction. It avoids the complicated technical details of the procedures and uses examples of their application for the most common eyesight problems as well as some of the more complex ones that have recently been successfully treated with advances in instrumentation and techniques."

Dr Richard C. Troutman, MD DSc(Hon) FACS FRCOphth
Founder of the *International Society of Refractive Surgery*

"This book should be read by anyone contemplating having laser surgery performed and who wishes to understand what is current in this field of ophthalmology. It recognises the past and gives thought to what the future may hold in the use of technology, especially lasers, in the correction of visual problems."

Professor Frank Martin, AM
Chairman of the Board of the Children's Medical Research Foundation
Past President and council member of The Royal Australian and New Zealand College of Ophthalmologists (RANZCO)

The Naked Eye

A.K.A. Publishing

The NAKED EYE

How the revolution of laser surgery has unshackled the human eye

G.S *Dr Gerard Sutton*

M.L *Dr Michael Lawless*

For further resources and the latest updates on laser eye surgery, visit our website, www.thenakedeyebook.com

First published 2013
Revised edition 2015

Published by
A.K.A. Publishing Pty Limited
303 Edgecliff Road
Woollahra 2025
Sydney, Australia

PO Box 2135
Strawberry Hills
NSW 2012
Australia

Phone 1300 69 78 67
Fax 1300 55 44 61
Email admin@akapublishing.com.au
Web www.akapublishing.com.au

ISBN 978-0-9872039-4-6
Editor Graeme Leslie Brosnan
Research Audrey Molloy
Cover Lauren Haire
Printed in Australia by Focus Print Group

Illustrations pages 22, 29, 41, 51, 87, 101, 123 Richard Wilkinson
All other illustrations Mark Erickson
Image page 78 reprinted with kind permission from the American Academy of Ophthalmology
Image page 85 reprinted with kind permission from Bruce Beresford
Image page 130 reprinted with kind permission from Professor John Marshall
Images page 53 and 54 reprinted with kind permission from Zeiss

the naked eye ~

the human eye, unassisted
by an optical instrument,
such as a telescope,
microscope, or spectacles…

CONTENTS

FEATURES

FOREWORD

Despite my gratitude to Dr Gerard Sutton for the laser eye surgery he performed on me around ten years ago, I approached his invitation to write a brief foreword to his co-written book about the subject with a feeling of dread, expecting to find the work about as exciting as listening to an Australian parliamentary broadcast or watching a Superhero movie. I was surprised to find myself engrossed.

Firstly, I found the history of laser eye surgery – a very recent history – to be fascinating, especially as the two pioneers of the process were working under relatively primitive conditions; Fyodorov in Russia, and Barraquer in Colombia. I remember being in London some years ago when Fyodorov had organised a Russian ship, replete with eye surgeons, to be parked in the Channel, presumably out of reach of government authorities. At that time the operation had not been officially approved and was categorised along with the Mexican witch doctors who offer cancer "cures". The more intrepid Brits with eye problems visited in fairly large numbers, I'm told, hopefully on days when the sea was calm, as the procedure is a delicate one, preferably not performed when the patient is unstable.

This book, by Dr Lawless and Dr Sutton, is written, mercifully, in layman's language and should answer the questions and allay the fears of those who are convinced that (a) there is a chance of blindness resulting from the operation (b) the operation has a chance of failure even without blindness resulting (c) the operation is painful and (d) the eyes are removed from the socket while the horrified patient is awake.

Speaking from personal experience with the calm and reassuring Dr Sutton, a master of the bedside manner, I can vouch that none of the above fears are valid. At the time of my visit to the practice I was wearing bifocals, having failed miserably with contact lenses. (I used to spend hours trying to get them into my eyes and finally thought of laser eye surgery after dropping the hundredth pair down the washbasin). Dr Sutton and his team examined my eyes thoroughly and I was told that the ideal solution was for one eye to be set for distance vision and the other for reading. This alarmed me initially but I was assured it is quite common and that "the brain adjusts so that there is no problem". Despite worries about the capability of my own brain I gave Dr Sutton the go-ahead.

A week or so after the operation I went to renew my driver's licence. The lady at the counter, looking at my application, said "It says here you need to wear glasses". "Not any more", I replied suavely. She pulled out an eye-chart and told me to read the bottom line. I read it so fluently that she looked dubious, convinced I had somehow managed to sneak a look at the chart and memorised it. On film sets now I have noticed the crew look on with bewilderment as, at age 73, my eye goes from the actors in front of the camera to the script in my hand without any pause, hesitation – or glasses.

I have recommended a number of people to Dr Sutton over the years, including my daughter, Trilby. At twenty-one she was wearing glasses so thick that she was actually legally blind. I went with her to the operation and sat beside her. The procedure took only a couple of minutes. She had to wear dark glasses (standard practice) for the remainder of that day. The next morning she woke in astonishment. Her vision was now perfect. She is now twenty-seven and this is still the case. The operation literally changed her life.

Bruce Beresford

Film Director, *Mao's Last Dancer, Driving Miss Daisy*

INTRODUCTION

If you want a book that explains all the pros and cons of laser eye surgery in an unbiased manner, in a language that you can understand and, as a result, make a decision as to whether or not this is for you, then you have found it.

This book is unique in that it is not the usual textbook whereby doctors massage their egos by bombarding the reader with complex and often irrelevant clinical information, and compound this further by intimidating you with the unnecessary technical language of ophthalmology. In crystal-clear and precise language it delivers all the information that anyone requires prior to considering laser eye surgery. Even as an expert in this field, I sometimes think that all the acronyms for vision correction procedures such as PRK, LASIK, LASEK and ASLA are entries in a secret competition between ophthalmologists and the military to see who can produce the least understandable combinations of letters. Ophthalmologists have a reputation amongst doctors for using words that even other doctors don't understand. However, the utmost attention has been paid throughout this book, through its jargon-free approach, to make sure that the lay reader understands everything.

This book is written by two special doctors who represent the very best of Australian medicine and who, at the same time, have achieved rightful positions of leadership in the international world of ophthalmology. Michael Lawless has played a major role in the International Society of Refractive Surgery and was the first ophthalmologist to really appreciate that the tests we carry out in clinics - e.g. reading the letter chart - are in reality hopeless measures in terms of determining the quality of vision after laser eye surgery. He designed a very special questionnaire rapidly adopted throughout the world to truly measure the quality of visual life before and after laser eye surgery. For the first time, patients actually had a say and could provide feedback as to how clear their vision really was in terms of this surgery.

Gerard Sutton realised that a major problem in the first technique in the early days of vision correction surgery was a transient loss of clarity of the cornea. He went on to carry out research which removed this problem and which has had profound implications for our understanding of wound-healing in all parts of the eye. The innovation, open-mindedness and clear thinking of these two individuals are the secrets of the future success of this volume.

Michael and Gerard have a great advantage in putting this text together in that they were two of the early pioneers in this field, having been there almost from the beginning. As a result they know personally all the major players who contributed as pioneers, and have lived through the history and development of vision correction surgery. They also jointly possess the ability to assimilate technical information in a rapidly changing field with the powers of discrimination to determine between good and bad advances. They have shared their considered opinions in the various chapters of this volume and have done so with their own remarkable brands of humour. By stamping their personalities on every page of this book they allow the reader to view the behind-the-scenes trials and tribulations that went on to perfect the most successful form of surgery in all fields of medicine. Their own contributions are immense and cannot be over-emphasised and are greatly appreciated by both their peers and their patients. I consider it a great honour to be invited to write this introduction and commend the book to you as I'm sure you will enjoy it as much as I did, and you will certainly use it as a lifelong reference for laser eye surgery for both yourself and all your friends interested in this field.

Professor John Marshall

Moorfields Eye Hospital, London, August 2013

THE NAKED EYE

One day in 1974, a 15 year old boy presented as a patient at an eye clinic in Moscow. His problem was unusual. He'd fallen from his bicycle and some pieces of glass had gone into one eye. For whatever reason, the boy received no medical treatment and although he appeared to have recovered, he now complained that one eye was 'different' to the other. It was presumed that the glass had damaged the cornea of one eye and, as it had been untreated, now affected his vision.

The doctor who treated him, Svyatoslav Fyodorov, examined the boy's eyes, and what he saw was to lead to the greatest revolution in eye surgery in hundreds of years. One eye, the boy's uninjured eye, was still short-sighted. The other eye, which had been cut by the piece of glass externally, had healed with a scar, yet incredibly the optical error had been fixed. He was no longer short-sighted in this eye. Fyodorov realised that the glass cut to the cornea had healed in a certain way that had repaired the short-sightedness in that eye. From this Fyodorov developed a new surgical technique and went on to make some of the greatest advances in the field of vision correction surgery.

Even though the evolution of laser vision correction is a truly fascinating story, there has been very little written about it. It is a mere fifty years since the first vision correction procedures were performed by José Barraquer in Colombia. But since then, vision correction surgery has had a turbulent history. The famous words of French physiologist, Claude Bernard, are very apt for this story: "The science of life is a superb and dazzlingly lighted hall which may be reached only by passing through a long and ghastly kitchen." Over the course of the past fifty years, a steady procession of pioneering doctors have stuck their necks out and risked their reputations to bring us closer to that nirvana for so many people – the ability to see with the naked eye – *without* corrective eyewear i.e. glasses and contact lenses. The entire story has played out across the globe, from Japan to Colombia, from Britain to Russia and the USA.

Both of us were, as young men, drawn to the exciting things which were happening in the world of ophthalmology. A lot has happened since that fifteen-year-old boy walked into Fyodorov's surgery, and we'd like to share that with you – particularly the advances of the last five years. Within our life-times, these extraordinary doctors around the world have advanced the field of vision correction surgery, often through very rocky territory, until we have reached the pinnacle of progress, today's procedures which, in the right hands and for the carefully chosen candidate, are the epitome of modern science – fabulously safe, predictable and accurate.

We feel very fortunate to be continuing the work of those brave ophthalmologists who set out to cure this age-old problem. We have interfaced with some of the biggest players in the history of the procedures and we have been privileged to be involved in setting new standards in surgical techniques, raising the bar to an all-time high in terms of safety.

If, like many people, you've noticed that your eyesight isn't what it used to be, this book should give you a better understanding of the surgical procedures currently available to reduce or eliminate your dependence on glasses. Of course this isn't meant to be a do-it-yourself or a self-diagnosis book. Nor does it constitute an informed consent for surgery. Each person deserves their own unique vision correction plan to achieve the best possible outcome and it is absolutely imperative that you discuss your particular situation with your doctor.

There are many misconceptions and myths about laser surgery and laser surgeons, one being that we are *against* spectacles. Almost *everyone* will require spectacles at some stage of their life – if not for distance vision then certainly for reading vision from mid-life onwards. Current life expectancy is heading for ninety years in developed countries, so you can expect to need reading glasses for half your life. In addition to this, we are seeing an epidemic of short-sightedness, particularly in East Asia, with recent studies showing 80-90% of their school leavers being short-sighted.[1] But it wasn't always like this. As you will read in the next chapter, short-sightedness is thought to be a fairly recent phenomenon – as is middle-age and its associated deterioration in near vision. Spectacles are currently the default solution for these eye conditions and while many people are happy to wear glasses if they need to, for some people (ourselves included) it is the *complete dependence* on glasses that is unacceptable. What has happened in the past decade is that a revolution has taken place in the many solutions available to provide freedom from glasses for everyday activities. Some of us may look back on the era of spectacle-wearing as an eyesight solution in the same way that we now fondly look back at the horse and cart as a mode of transport. With laser vision correction we are entering an exciting new era in medical science. And we'd like you to be part of that story.

What has happened in the past decade is that a revolution has taken place in the many solutions available to provide freedom from glasses for everyday activities.

We wanted to create a book that was accessible to everyone, as well as being of interest to the prospective patient, and also something that industry professionals may find helpful in their practices. Whilst this book is clinically correct, we have avoided as much as we can complicated explanations and technical jargon. Also, it's a dip-in dip-out book and not necessarily meant to be read from cover to cover. You can pick and choose what interests you. This book will tell you the story of vision correction science – where it has come from, where it is today and perhaps what the future may hold. It will also enlighten you on what is involved in having laser eye surgery today. You'll learn about the various procedures available, gain some insight into the history of eye surgery, and hopefully be entertained along the way.

We trust that, having read this book, you will be better informed as to the range of choices available, how they work, and what you can anticipate if you have a vision correction procedure. Also, we hope that our book tells you things you never knew, introduces you to some of the wonderful stories of our patients, and opens your eyes to the world of ophthalmology.

Dr Michael Lawless | Professor Gerard Sutton

M.L

A REMARKABLE INSTRUMENT

I see trees of green, red roses too,
I see 'em bloom for me and you,
And I think to myself, what a wonderful world.

As you read the evocative lyrics of Louis Armstrong's wonderful song you are using the most incredible device in the human body. Vision is part of the bedrock of our daily lives and yet most of us take it for granted. As ophthalmologists we specialise in looking after people's eyes and wanted to share with you some of the fascinating history of vision science and vision correction surgery and the interesting characters that made it happen.

Arguably Australia's most famous ophthalmologist was Professor Fred Hollows, who, in the 1960s and 70s, conducted tests that recorded the best vision anywhere in the world. When he journeyed to the Australian outback and put Aboriginal people in front of an eye chart he couldn't believe the results. Short-sightedness was unknown in Aboriginal people and in those eyes without disease they achieved the best test results ever recorded. It was such an unexpected outcome. It is believed that the Australian Aboriginal people lived virtually in isolation from the rest of the world for at least 40,000 years. During that time their eyes evolved excellent distance vision, which was ideal for the Australian climate and geography and their hunter-gatherer life-style. They developed better distance vision and better quality of vision than people in other parts of the world – people with more 'modern' lifestyles living in agrarian societies where there was division of labour and a lot more close work involved. In that sense, Hollows' data on the Australian Aboriginals is the best understanding we have of how the eye might have been for our species – Homo sapiens – before modern times. When Governor Phillip and the First Fleet landed in Sydney in 1788, the 'savages' they encountered had far superior vision to theirs.

The Aboriginals had incredibly sharp vision for hunting and seeing in the distance over large areas. They had no refractive error – no short-sightedness or astigmatism – it just didn't exist in their people.[2]

Superior vision was once the difference between life and death. And for most species it still is. It conferred a great advantage on humans in pre-modern times because we had what is known as predator vision – and we still have this today. The eyes of all living creatures can be divided basically into two sorts. There are creatures that eat other creatures – the predators, and creatures that get eaten – the prey. That's basically what it comes down to. The eyes of predators and prey are fundamentally different. For example, the human eye is a bit like an eagle's eye so we can see very sharply at long distances. And we have very good depth perception, so we can see objects in 3D. But we don't have particularly good peripheral vision or night vision. In contrast, an antelope (or any creature that gets preyed upon) doesn't have very good depth perception but what it does have is great peripheral vision so it can see something approaching and then run away or hide. When our ancestors stood up millions of years ago – evolving from apes to early man – they could see a long way. They could see prey. This was an evolutionary advantage.

Another evolutionary advantage was our ability to continuously see stationary objects. You cannot see it happening, but your eye is never perfectly still. Even when your eye is staring – fixated on an object – small, jerky, involuntary movements called micro-saccades occur every few seconds. If we go back millions of years to how eyes evolved, this is to do with how the brain actually detects movement. (It was very useful to be able to tell something moving from something still because that something could be food. Or we could be food for it…). We have specialised nerve cells called 'edge detectors' built into our retina and our visual cortex. They 'fire' when they detect the edge of an object and we 'detect' it. A scientist called Troxler noticed that if we stabilise all eye movements and stare at a non-moving image it will fade from view after several seconds. However, our micro-saccades cause the image of the object we are looking at to 'jump' slightly on our retina so we can continue to observe it without fading.

Reptile's eyes can't continuously see something unless that something is moving, a fact which is played out in the movie *Jurassic Park* ... "Don't move! He can't see us if we don't move." (Incidentally, it is actually believed that T-Rex *could* see stationary objects because of the size of the visual cortex of his brain and the placement of his eyes, but that doesn't make for good cinema...). This is certainly true of a frog's eyes. A frog will starve to death surrounded by food if that food is not moving. If something is insect-sized and it moves then a frog will eat it. But our eyes, like the eyes of many mammals, *can* continuously detect stationary objects because of those tiny eye movements – the micro-saccades. Later, in this book we'll talk more about how the laser surgeon deals with this continuous eye movement during a vision correction procedure.

Even if you have no genetically passed-on eyesight problems, as you advance in age your near vision will deteriorate to the extent that you need something to compensate for it. In evolutionary terms, this is a fairly recent phenomenon. In pre-modern times (50,000 to 10,000 years ago, before the advent of agriculture), it is estimated that life-expectancy was 54 years of age. This is based on data from hunter-gatherer populations.[3]

As life expectancy increased rapidly over time we faced the problem of living through the latter decades of life without clear near vision. Sometime around the year 1000 AD it was noticed that curved glass could magnify the size of objects viewed through that glass. By about the year 1200 AD two pieces of magnifying glass had been attached to a frame and worn as glasses.

Apart from refinements in grinding and developing the lenses, glasses were used in essentially the same way for the rest of the millennium. Nothing much changed for almost 800 years. And then in the relatively brief period from the 1950s to today, there were the most amazing advances in technology and surgical procedures in ophthalmology. In 1949 hard contact lenses made from Perspex were invented.

These were designed to sit on the cornea – the front surface of the eye – and could be worn for up to sixteen hours a day, but not without adverse effects on the eyes over time. Over the following decades the materials were improved and soft lenses were introduced. In the very first Sean Connery James Bond film, *Dr No* (1962) one of the villains from *Spectre* appears wearing soft contact lenses. The arrival of the soft contact lens was a boon for many as they were more comfortable than hard lenses, but when you took them out, you still had the original problem. Surgical intervention was the only way to permanently improve a person's vision and what is now regarded as the pivotal moment in ophthalmology happened by accident, because of an accident.

Svyatoslav Nikolayevich Fyodorov, an ophthalmologist in Moscow, treated a fifteen-year-old boy who'd fallen from his bicycle and had had some pieces of glass in one eye. What Fyodorov saw and what he did led to the greatest revolution in eye surgery in hundreds of years. Fyodorov realised that the eye's surface had healed in a certain way, which had repaired the short-sightedness in that eye. From this Fyodorov developed a new surgical technique and went on to make some of the greatest advances in the field of corrective surgery.

If you're reading this book then you probably want to know more about laser vision correction. In order to do so you need to understand a little bit about the eye itself and how it works. The eye is one of the most amazing organs in our body. It is responsible for our sense of sight and is constructed of materials not found anywhere else in our bodies. The rest of our tissues are made up of bones, muscles, blood vessels and various kinds of connective tissue. However, our eyes have *clear* structures i.e. the cornea and the crystalline lens, which allow light to pass straight through them and onto the retina at the back of our eye. The eye is almost like something artificial that has been put in the body because it has these clear tissues that are not present anywhere else. But the eye is also an organ, so although it resembles an optical instrument, it is actually flesh and blood and prone to a range of diseases and infections.

Think of the eye as being like a camera. The eyelid is like the lens cap and when you open it you see the cornea, which is like the main lens of the camera. What you see is captured at the back of the eye by

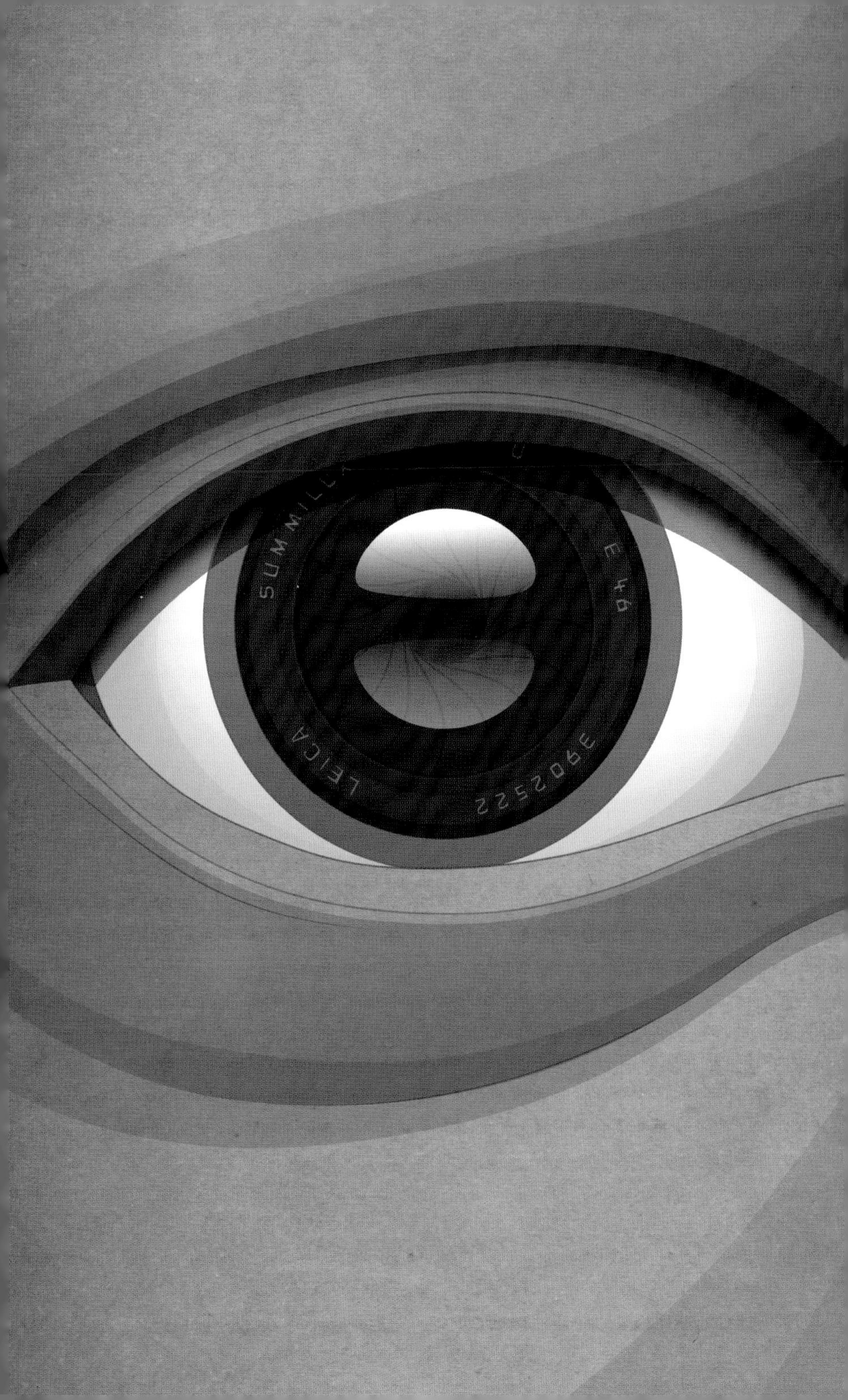
LEICA
E 46

the retina, which acts like the film in a camera. From there it is sent to the 'lab', the visual cortex of our brain, situated right at the back of our head in the occipital lobes. This is where the image is 'developed' and we can make sense of the world we see.

One of the most remarkable things about the eye is the transparency of several of its structures. How it happens to be transparent is a fascinating subject.

Light travels in waves of a certain wavelength. The way the cornea and lens of your eye are constructed allows for light waves to simply pass right through them. The cornea and lens are constructed of collagen fibres arranged in a very orderly fashion – much like very orderly stacked drainpipes. The wavelength of light is such that it literally weaves its way through the orderly spaces between the fibres and passes right through. If the cornea or lens gets damaged through eye disease or accident, the collagen fibres lose their orderly arrangement and we develop a scar and light can no longer pass through.

The collagen fibres make up almost the entire thickness of the cornea apart from a thin layer of cells at the front (the epithelium) and the back (the endothelium) and two membranes separating these thin layers from the main body (the stroma) of the cornea. The natural lens within the eye (which is called the crystalline lens) is also made up of neatly ordered collagen fibres and has an outer layer called the capsule. ●

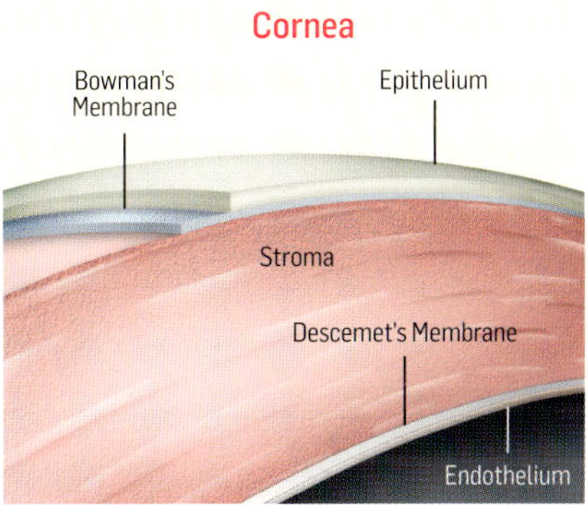

The cornea consists of five layers

G.S

HOW THE EYE SEES

It is a simple fact that light changes direction when it moves from one transparent medium to another. If we look at a drinking straw in a glass of water it seems to bend, and objects underwater appear to be in a different place to where they really are.

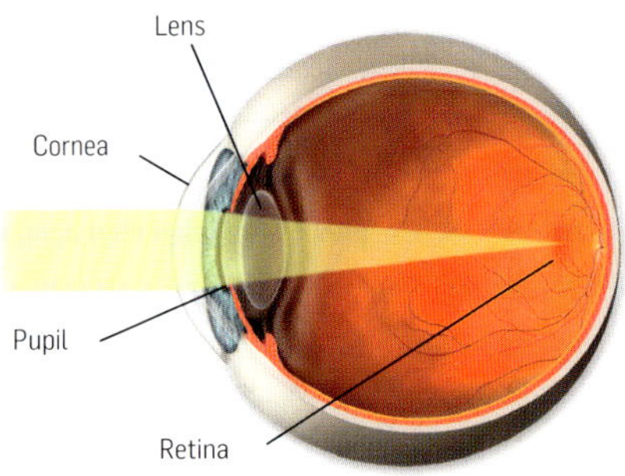

The clearly focused eye

When light moves from air to water it changes direction. As the cornea, crystalline lens and various fluids within the eye all bend light in a very similar way, the main change in direction occurs when the light passes through your cornea. If your eye is optically perfect, light from distance objects reaches the front surface of the eye and is bent so that it comes to a clear focus on the retina at the back of your eye. This requires the curvature of your cornea to be precisely in tune with the length of your eye (from cornea to retina).

However, if the eye is longer or shorter than this ideal or if the cornea is more or less curved, then the image will not be in clear focus. There are four main conditions which are usually diagnosed in these situations: myopia, hyperopia, astigmatism and presbyopia.

Short-sightedness – or **myopia**. Here the cornea is *too steeply curved* (relative to the length of the eye) to focus the image clearly onto your retina and vision is blurred in the distance. An advantage of short-sightedness is the ability to see up close without spectacles. Short-sightedness commonly develops as you grow and typically is detected in childhood or adolescence. It may progress into your twenties or in extreme cases even later.

Long-sightedness – or **hyperopia**. Here the cornea is *too flat* (relative to the length of the eye) to focus the image clearly onto your retina. Your distance vision will be better than your near vision, although as you get older your distance vision will also become blurred. While your natural lens can compensate for some degree of long-sightedness when you are younger (keeping you out of glasses for a while), long-sightedness is the most common reason that glasses are prescribed for full-time use in mid to later life.

Astigmatism usually occurs in combination with either short- or long-sightedness. Here the cornea is more curved in one contour than the other, resulting in vision that can be blurred for both distance and close up. It requires a more complex correction which is not usually a problem for glasses but can be a problem in obtaining satisfactory vision with contact lenses. Astigmatism is usually not an impediment to a surgical vision correction solution.

If you are long-sighted, short-sighted or have astigmatism, you may be suitable for a vision correction procedure, to either eliminate or greatly reduce your dependence on glasses or contact lenses. Whether you are suitable for vision

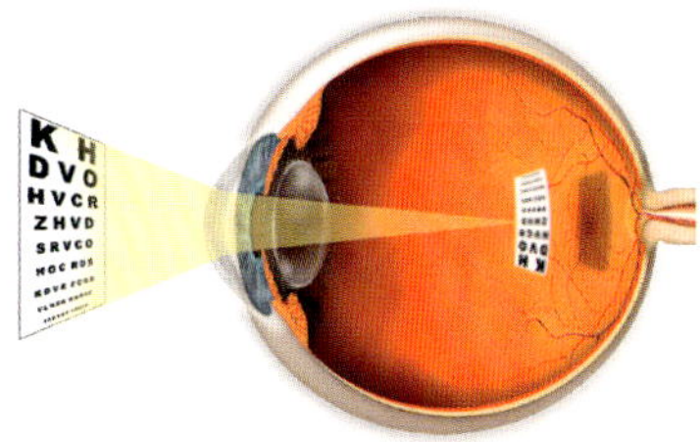

Short-sightedness or myopia

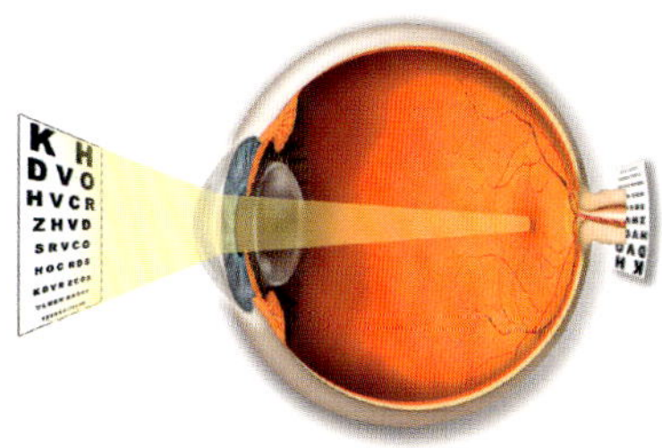

Long-sightedness or hyperopia

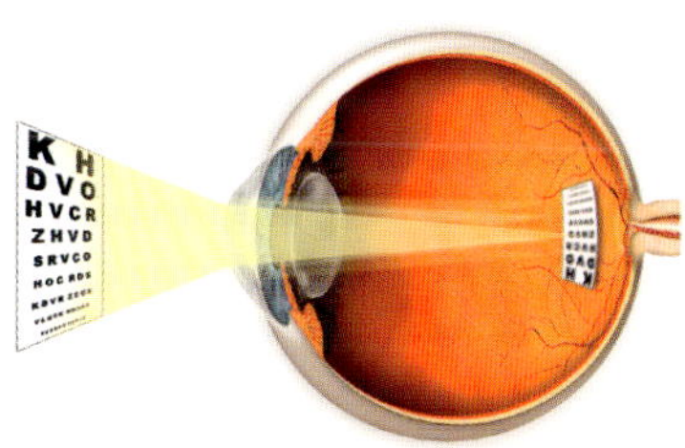

Astigmatism

correction surgery depends on a number of factors – not just your glasses prescription.

Presbyopia comes from the Greek word *presby*, meaning 'elder' and *opia*, meaning 'sightedness'. Presbyopia is a fact of life for all of us. Even when you are clearly focused for distance vision, the natural lens within your eye is constantly working to fine-tune your focus from distance to near – in much the same way as the zoom lens on a camera. However, as you approach your mid-forties your natural lens is no longer able to work as hard and your near vision becomes blurred. This is called presbyopia. Good lighting can help for a while but it is not long before you need the help of reading glasses to see small print. If you are already wearing glasses or contact lenses for distance then you will need to change to multifocal or bifocal lenses so that you can see in the distance *and* close up. Short-sighted people often just take off their glasses to read, as they naturally have good close vision.

If you have presbyopia, objects that are near you, such as a computer, smart phone or menu will be difficult to see. ●

See *Presbyopia and Vision Correction*, page 32, and *The Beauty of Blended Vision*, page 82.

G.S 20/20 VISION

An adult with perfect vision can read the small letters of the eye-test chart at six metres (or twenty feet, as in 20/20 vision). These letters are very small — right at the limit of what the human eye can see — and are roughly a little under a centimetre in height.

I wish I'd caught a fish for every person who's ever asked me to explain 20/20 vision (or 6/6 metric as Australian ophthalmologists and optometrists refer to it). I guess it's something that everyone's heard of, but no one has a clue what it means. So here goes: The first 20 is simple. It is just the distance from your eye to where the letter chart is – 6 metres in Australia (or 20 feet in the US – hence the 20). All ophthalmologists' and optometrists' consulting rooms are designed to have a distance of exactly 20 feet between the patient's eyes and the letter chart. That's why they almost always use a mirror. When you look at the letter chart reflected in a mirror the room only needs to be 10 feet long instead of 20 feet. Much more affordable for premises in the High Street!

The second 20 (in 20/20) is a bit trickier to explain. If you can read the letters on the 20/20 line of the vision chart at 20 feet then you are seeing the smallest letters that the average adult can read with a fully healthy eye. (In fact, most human eyes have a visual potential of slightly better than 20/20). In this way you can think of 20/20 as meaning 20/normal. Some people can see those letters without glasses, so their **uncorrected** vision is 20/20. This is usually what most people want to achieve from laser vision correction; 20/20 vision with the naked eye.

Others can only see those little letters with corrective lenses in place – we call this their **best-corrected** vision. The average adult with a healthy eye should be able to read 20/20 with or without corrective lenses. If their eye is not healthy, for example due to a cataract or macular degeneration, then they will not be capable of reading the letters on the 20/20 line of the vision chart, **even with** their corrective lenses. They might have a best corrected vision of 20/40. This means that they can see from 20 feet away what a healthy eye could see from 40 feet away. Some people have very sharp vision – better than average. They may be able to read even smaller letters than most. Their vision might be 20/15, meaning that they can read from 20 feet away what most people can only read from 15 feet away.

20/20 vision is considered the best level of vision for humans. So if you're in the 20/20 category and feeling pleased with yourself, think about this: The tiny letters you can see on the bottom of the chart from 20 feet, a wedge-tail eagle can see from 100 feet – its vision is the same as ours at **five times** the distance. (If a human could see as well as an eagle they would have 20/4 vision, meaning that from 20 feet they could read letters that the average adult with a healthy eye and the best corrective lens could only read from a distance of 4 feet). However, I should also explain that the eagle has a different kind of eye as well as a different way that it is hardwired to their brain. So, now you know. ●

M.L

THE ANCIENTS

"People's desire to get out of their glasses is not a recent phenomenon. They have been thinking about alternatives to wearing glasses for hundreds of years. Why? Because, for the majority of people, it feels like a handicap. It is rarely a cosmetic issue. The issue is that if you wear glasses, you are dependent on something that is like a crutch. It is like having hearing loss. You can hear with a hearing aid, but you would prefer not to have the hearing aid."

Dr Michael Lawless

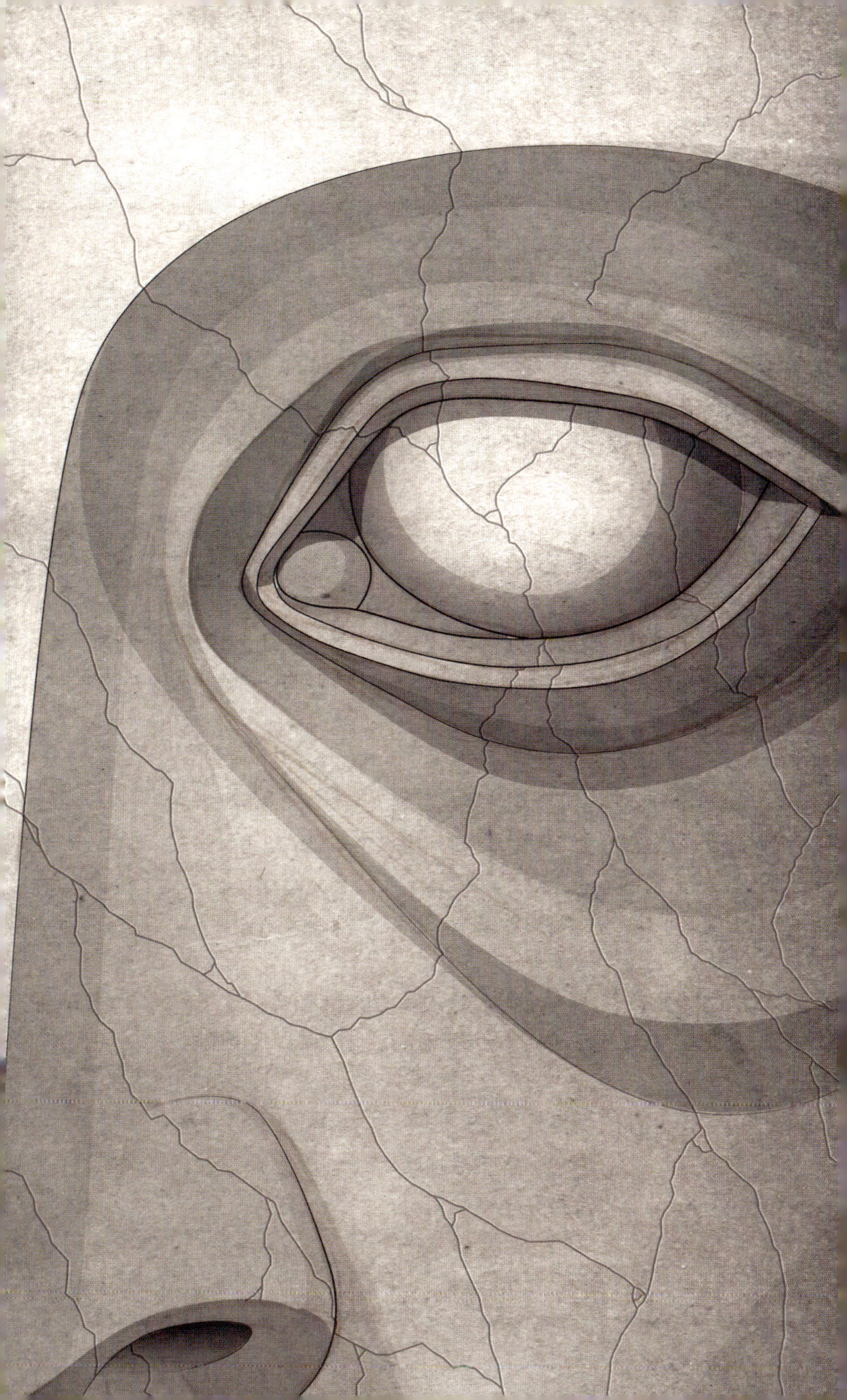

The eye is one of surgery's oldest interests. We know from the Babylonians that some form of eye surgery was happening at least as far back as 1750 BC.

One of their kings, Hammurabi, enacted a code of 282 laws which governed a wide cross-section of issues including family relationships, inheritance, divorce, legal responsibilities and penalties for breaching the code. No 215 states, "If a surgeon has operated with the bronze lancet on a patrician for a serious injury, and has cured him, or has removed with a bronze lancet a cataract for a patrician, and has cured his eye, he shall take ten shekels of silver." This is the earliest known reference to eye surgery and confirms that the Babylonians used lens depression for the treatment of cataracts almost 4,000 years ago.

The first recorded surgical technique for treating cataracts, known as 'couching', was documented by the Indian physician, Sushruta, in his book, **Compendium**, in 800 BC. He describes an operation in which a curved needle is used to push the "opaque phlegmatic matter" out of the way of vision. The "phlegm" was then blown out through the nose, or pushed into the back of the eye. Sushruta recommended using breast milk to irrigate the eye during the procedure to assist the recovery process. What the Indian physician does not mention in his **Compendium** is that although the patient could see again, their vision was limited and would only deteriorate. Also, the risk of complications leading to permanent loss of vision was considerable.

There are no surviving records of any new eye-surgery techniques for the next 800 years until the Roman era. Physicians working in Ancient Rome recorded in 29 AD various remedies for cataracts, short-sightedness and conjunctivitis. For the treatment of cataract, Roman physicians used a range of variously sized needles, which were carefully inserted into the eye to break up the cataract into smaller particles. The sharp end of the needle would assist in the surgical process, whilst the blunt end would be used to cauterise the wound. Peculiarly, this was accompanied by administering blows to the patient's head to assist the extraction process.

Then, approximately 800 years later, in the 10th century, the Persian physician Muhammad ibn Zakariya al-Razi, detailed a cataract procedure where the lens was removed using a bronze oral suction instrument. Zakariya al-Razi generously attributed the procedure to a 2nd century Greek physician, Antyllus. When performing this operation, the physician needed "an assistant with an extraordinary lung capacity" to suck the lens out of the eye.

This suction procedure was also described by the Iraqi ophthalmologist Ammar ibn Ali in his **Choice of Eye Diseases**. In this 10th century work, ibn

Ali also provided case histories of a number of patients whom he claimed to have treated successfully.

It was to be another 800 years before French medical practitioner Jacques Daviel successfully extracted cataracts from the eye. Dr Daviel set up an ophthalmology practice in 1728 and performed the first extra-capsular cataract extraction in 1747. This procedure involved the removal of almost the whole of the patient's natural lens, leaving just the back of the lens' very thin capsule (or skin) intact. The patient's natural lens was manually removed through a centimetre-wide incision in the front surface of the eye. This was acknowledged as being the first significant advance in cataract surgery since couching became known over 2,000 years earlier.

The more things change, the more they stay the same. When ophthalmologist and African mission worker, Dr Wendy Hofman was conducting a clinic in Gabon (West Africa) in 2010, she came face-to-face with a patient who had undergone the ancient cataract surgical procedure known as 'couching'. The patient seen by Dr Hofman advised that he had been to a 'medical practitioner' in Pointe Noir in the Republic of the Congo who boasted he could do cataract surgery without any surgical instruments, let alone an operating room. This sounded ideal to the patient, but after the procedure he had eye pain and worsening blindness. When examined by Dr Hofman in the hospital in Gabon, he was blind to the level of only being able to differentiate light from dark. His eye pressure was very elevated, and his optic nerve almost completely destroyed. Unfortunately, there was little they could do for this patient apart from pain relief. ●

PRESBYOPIA AND VISION CORRECTION

The word presbyopia comes from the Greek word presby, meaning 'elder' and opia, meaning 'sightedness'. Presbyopia is the inability of the eye to focus up close as you get older. If you are thirty years old and have normal distance vision then you don't have to wear glasses to read. But if you are over fifty and you have normal distance vision then you most probably need to wear glasses to read because you have presbyopia – a loss of elasticity in the natural lens within the eye that affects everyone as they get older.

Blended Vision

If you are over fifty years old and you don't want to wear reading glasses then there are a number of options to consider in developing a vision correction plan. Sometimes we recommend a laser vision correction procedure on your cornea and aim for **blended vision** (see *The Beauty of Blended Vision*, page 82) where we make the dominant eye really good for distance and the other eye a bit short-sighted deliberately. It doesn't address the primary issue of the loss of elasticity in your natural lens but improves your ability to read close up. **Blended vision** is not perfect but it is a practical and straightforward solution for many people. Others achieve blended vision with their contact lenses as they get older – they have one eye clear for distance and the other a bit better for reading.

Blended vision works because despite what you may think, much of the time we are not in fact seeing equally with both eyes. Even though you have both eyes open, it may surprise you to know that one eye – the dominant eye – does more of the work. Blended vision leverages off this fact by making the dominant eye clear for distance (in the vast majority of cases), whilst the non-dominant eye is reset to allow it to read close up. There is some compromise. You will always see better at a particular distance if both eyes are working together, but some people are very willing to make that compromise so that they are less dependent on reading glasses.

Blended vision sometimes occurs naturally. A few lucky people are naturally a bit short-sighted in one eye but have good distance vision in the other. If you have grown up with it, it is easy because your brain understands very clearly what this is about. For the rest of the population who might be considering surgical intervention to achieve blended vision, you can demonstrate what it will be like by doing a contact lens trial. You can easily test-drive the effect and determine if blended vision is a sensible endpoint for you. In terms of vision correction surgery, blended vision can be achieved with either a laser vision correction procedure on your cornea (see *LASIK, ASLA and SMILE Laser*, page 52) or, increasingly common in the over fifty-fives, a lens replacement procedure (see *Laser Lens Surgery*, page 90).

Lens replacement surgery is commonly used to correct short-sightedness, long-sightedness, astigmatism and reading vision problems, especially in people over the age of fifty-five. It is often a more suitable procedure than LASIK, ASLA or SMILE for this age group – especially if you are very short-sighted or long-sighted. ●

CASE STUDY*

ROBERT KAYE, OPTOMETRIST, AGE 75

Like many people, I first experienced signs of short-sightedness in my early high school days. Objects in the distance were out of focus and blurry, particularly at night. My parents took me to the local optometrist who prescribed glasses.

* Due to patient confidentiality and privacy considerations, some patient details have been altered for the purposes of this book. Also, some of the case studies presented are a composite of cases we have seen. However, the medical histories, surgical experiences and results are real.

I decided this procedure was not for someone like me who has a risk-averse personality. I was not keen to be a guinea pig.

As my short-sightedness (myopia) progressively worsened it started to affect my sporting activities – mainly cricket and rugby – and this really hit home when I was dropped from the 'firsts' to the 'seconds' in each. Head protection was not as common or as advanced at that time, so wearing glasses for cricket without head-gear was not considered safe. The optometrist recommended hard contact lenses (soft lenses had not yet been invented). Hard lenses turned out to be uncomfortable, and it was a nuisance to carry spares and a cleaning kit. Because of this handicap I became less involved in sport during my university days, something I really regretted. At this point the Roads and Traffic Authority found that glasses were a legal requirement for my driving.

So, it was something of a coincidence that I studied optometry and after graduation became involved in a clinical practice, taking care of the visual needs of patients, many of whom had eye problems similar to mine.

I wore glasses for distance and near sight until about the age of forty-eight. It was then I noticed I could see better close-up without my glasses. I knew to expect this as a normal part of the ageing process. Also, I had obtained my private pilot's licence and was flying light aircraft for recreation.

About this time, radial keratotomy (known as The Russian Technique) became available for vision correction. However, following research – the hard way – neither Google nor laser vision correction had been invented – I decided this procedure was not for someone like me who has a risk-averse personality. I was not keen to be a guinea pig.

Working as an optometrist gave me access to the full range of contact lenses available and this enabled me to experiment with different forms of prescription without 'breaking the bank'. Soft contact lenses solved my problem of discomfort and allowed longer wearing time. Initially they were only available to correct the short-sighted part of my prescription, but I had astigmatism as well as myopia. I needed both parts to give the best vision. Fortunately, technology advanced and I was able to achieve satisfactory comfort and clear vision. By this time, age had caught up with my close work and I needed bifocals. I tried bifocal contact lenses but found these limited my working area and there were 'out of focus' patches. This compromise was not for me and I was unable to continue wearing soft contact lenses.

When I reached my sixties I realised cataracts were forming in both eyes. Things were becoming dimmer at night, street lights and car headlights were 'yellowish' and I had difficulty making out facial features, especially if the light was coming from behind the person. In my case the short-sightedness became worse; in fact my prescription almost doubled in one eye! I knew that not everyone has the same signs and symptoms, so I had this confirmed by an optometrist and later by an ophthalmologist. I was officially experiencing the symptoms of mild cataracts (cloudiness of the natural lenses within my eyes that comes on with age).

Like many of my patients I consulted Dr Google but found this information confusing and so decided to trust my ophthalmologist's advice.

Regrettably at this time I handed in my pilot's licence and instead continued my love of aviation by building a flight simulator. Walking and swimming were now more appropriate activities. The inconvenience of wearing multifocal glasses and tinted prescription sunglasses, supplemented by reading glasses, and the economics of the situation prompted me to think that it was time for the 'old' lenses that I was born with to be replaced. Like many of my patients I consulted Dr Google but found this information confusing and so decided to trust my ophthalmologist's advice. We discussed my expectations and needs and how this operation would impact my life.

Some of the options were: Did I want to be glasses-free? Did I want to have good distance vision without glasses but use a pair of readers for close work? What about computers? Did I want to have good computer and reading vision but wear glasses for distance? Did I want to have blended vision – one eye dominant for distance and the other eye used for close-up? Decisions, decisions ... it was even confusing for me as an optometrist!

I advised the surgeon that I didn't mind wearing glasses for some activities as long as I was not totally dependent on them – after all I had worn spectacles for most of my life – and they did support the vanity of hiding some facial ageing! Realistically, I would be content to wear 'ordinary' (but not 'thick') lenses for night driving and movies as well as occasional reading glasses for fine print if the lighting wasn't adequate. 'Could this be achieved for me?' We agreed on a blended vision plan which would aim to correct my short-sightedness and astigmatism and also allow me to maximise my independence from glasses for reading and computer work. This plan would fit in with my 'needs' and 'wants'. A date was fixed to do my right eye first, followed by my left eye six months later. (The usual protocol is to perform the procedures at least a week or two apart). The procedure was painless and in each case completed in a morning. The next day the clear shield was removed and the eye examined in the doctor's rooms. I was amazed how good the vision was at this early stage. This turned out to be suitable and convenient for my lifestyle.

Reflecting on the experience I think it's very important to let the surgeon know what your expectations are and be realistic. For some it may not be important to read the bottom line on the eye chart. There may need to be some compromise. Fifty years of working with people has taught me that many patients don't want to bother the surgeon and 'waste' their time with 'silly' questions. They find it difficult to know what to ask and often leave the consulting room with more questions than they went in with.

Now I am happy with the outcome. Although I'm still getting used to the blended vision, I am able to work at my computer without the need for spectacles, and daytime driving is back to what it was in my younger days. The convenience of being glasses-free for most of my working and leisure day makes me appreciate how lucky we are to have these procedures. Finally, my restored vision allowed me to re-apply for my recreational pilot's licence and I had great pleasure in fronting up to the Roads and Traffic Authority to have them remove the requirement to wear glasses while driving.

Intraocular Lenses

During lens replacement surgery (also called laser lens surgery) your natural lens is removed and replaced with a new artificial lens (also called an intraocular lens). There are a number of different designs of artificial lens to choose from. If you have astigmatism, we may put in a lens to correct your astigmatism. That would make your distance vision perfect, but you'd still need reading glasses because there is no elastic property to that type of artificial lens. Another option to consider is the *multifocal* intraocular lens. However, the terminology can be confusing. They are not multifocal in quite the same way as glasses can be multifocal. What multifocal intraocular lenses attempt to do is give you distance vision and reading vision as well as everything in between. They do that quite well for the right candidate, although there is always a slight compromise to the quality or crispness of your vision compared to how your own eyes worked before the onset of presbyopia.

What multifocal intraocular lenses attempt to do is give you distance vision and reading vision as well as everything in between.

If you are over fifty-five and you are having laser lens surgery or laser cataract surgery, you have to make a decision as to what matters most to you. If you're a bit pedantic and you want perfect distance vision and that's the thing that matters – perfect night vision, perfect clarity for distance – you are better off having implanted a non-multifocal artificial lens and making both eyes perfect for distance. This will mean you will have to wear a pair of glasses for reading. That might be the perfect solution for some personality types. Or, you might be one of those people who knows that their vision is not perfect anyway, so you don't *mind* a slight compromise in your quality of vision as long as you don't have to wear glasses at all after your procedure.

The only way to be reasonably certain of achieving that is to have a multifocal lens implanted in each eye. This is in a sense the opposite of blended vision – it makes both eyes exactly the same. The multifocal lens allows you to see in the distance and read, and also see the bits in between albeit at some slight cost in terms of quality of vision. For most people, this variation in quality of vision is almost unnoticeable, but for a person who might be an artist, an architect, or a particular personality type, that compromise needs to be carefully considered when deciding which sort of artificial lens to have put in. They are all good lenses of course, it's just that they all have pros and cons in terms of what they are doing for your eyes. This is where meticulous patient selection comes in. The right procedure for your eye depends not only on your spectacle prescription and age but also on your occupation, hobbies and even your personality. ●

CASE STUDY

Here is a typical scenario.

Eddie, a seventy-two year old retired lawyer comes in for a consultation. He's planning a big trip with his wife around Australia and he's just sick of his glasses. In his younger years Eddie had great vision and only started wearing glasses in his forties, just for reading at first, but gradually they became necessary for more and more activities until about ten years ago when he commenced full-time wear. He wears multifocals. A keen fisherman, he likes to cast off the rocks at Long Reef headland with a huge beach-caster and catch a few snapper. Also, he likes to race his little J24 yacht fairly aggressively around Pittwater and he is forever replacing his expensive glasses due to loss or corrosion from sea salt. With all this in mind Eddie's decided to take the plunge. He's a fairly relaxed fellow and open to any vision correction solution that will get him out of glasses for outdoors activities. However, he's fine with the idea of using a pair of readers for small print and he's even fine with the idea of glasses for occasional night driving or movies. So, here we have an ideal candidate for vision correction surgery, assuming his eyes are suitable!

Eddie's prescription is pretty straight-forward. He's long-sighted (about +3 for distance) and has presbyopia (about +5 for reading) and has nice thick corneas, so it's all looking good for LASIK. However, considering his age and the fact that his own natural lenses no longer give him any help with his reading vision, Eddie could alternatively have a vision correction procedure on his lens. When I look at his lenses, I notice they are actually quite cloudy and he admits that his optometrist had told him that there were cataracts developing in his eyes. But so far they hadn't bothered him too much. When we discuss it he acknowledges that he has noticed increased glare in sunlight and some difficulty seeing signs when driving, both classic symptoms of cataract.

Eddie's vision correction plan is a no-brainer. Basically, he needs cataract surgery. This will involve a micro-surgery technique to remove the cloudy material inside his natural lens and replace it with an artificial lens which is exactly tailored to his visual needs and will maximise his independence from glasses. This procedure is identical to the clear lens replacement surgery we do when there is no cataract present and the patient just wants spectacle independence.

In fact, if we consider modern cataract surgery under the umbrella of vision correction procedures, then it is by far the most frequently performed vision correction procedure in the world. Millions of cataract procedures are performed every year all around the globe. In the majority of cases, the patient not only gets rid of the cataract causing their cloudy vision, but they can also have their independence from glasses greatly improved by the surgery. We regularly see an elderly patient, who has depended on heavy spectacles their whole life, suddenly liberated from them when they have their cataracts out and a new intraocular lens put in their eyes. Sure, they may still have glasses for some elements of their life – usually for reading and sometimes also for driving – but their dependence on glasses is usually greatly reduced. This huge upside in having your lenses replaced is partly what has driven clear lens replacement, where a patient with a perfectly clear lens and no sign of a cataract elects to have their lenses replaced, simply to get rid of their glasses. There are other factors of course, including the improvements in the intraocular lenses available as well as the surgical techniques

We regularly see an elderly patient, who has depended on heavy spectacles their whole life, suddenly liberated from them when they have their cataracts out and a new intraocular lens put in their eyes.

which make a clear lens replacement a very valid option for the right candidate when choosing a vision correction plan for them.

The silver lining for Eddie is that because he has significant cataracts he will not only see a lot more sharply after surgery, but he will have less out-of-pocket costs as both Medicare and his private health fund partially cover the cost of cataract surgery. There will still be a gap but it is quite a bit less than he had budgeted for laser vision correction so he's pretty pleased with himself and we haven't even done the surgery yet!

The next step is an in-depth discussion with him about what type of vision will give him most independence from glasses. We look at this from every angle – his personality, his age, his glasses prescription, his hobbies and interests and after all that we decide to replace his natural lenses with multifocal artificial lenses (or intraocular lenses). This will give him good binocular vision for distance and near and because his vision is already slightly compromised by his developing cataracts he is very unlikely to be concerned by any slight compromise to visual quality caused by the multifocal optics of his new lenses.

We schedule surgery, with the eyes being treated one week apart. He can see 20/20 again for distance and near and so far has no need of glasses. He sent us a postcard from Broome saying he loves his newfound freedom from glasses and couldn't be happier with his outcome. They're the ones that make you smile!

Two things have converged to make lens replacement (laser lens surgery) a more sensible option than it would have been even ten years ago. One has been the ability to use a laser to replace several of the manual steps of the lens replacement surgical procedure. This has resulted in better predictability and outcomes for today's patients. The other reason is that the range and design of artificial lenses available to replace your natural lens has improved dramatically over the past ten years. These new generation artificial lenses mimic what your own lenses were like when you were thirty-five or forty years old. ●

For more surgical options to treat presbyopia see *Other Vision Correction Procedures*, page 104.

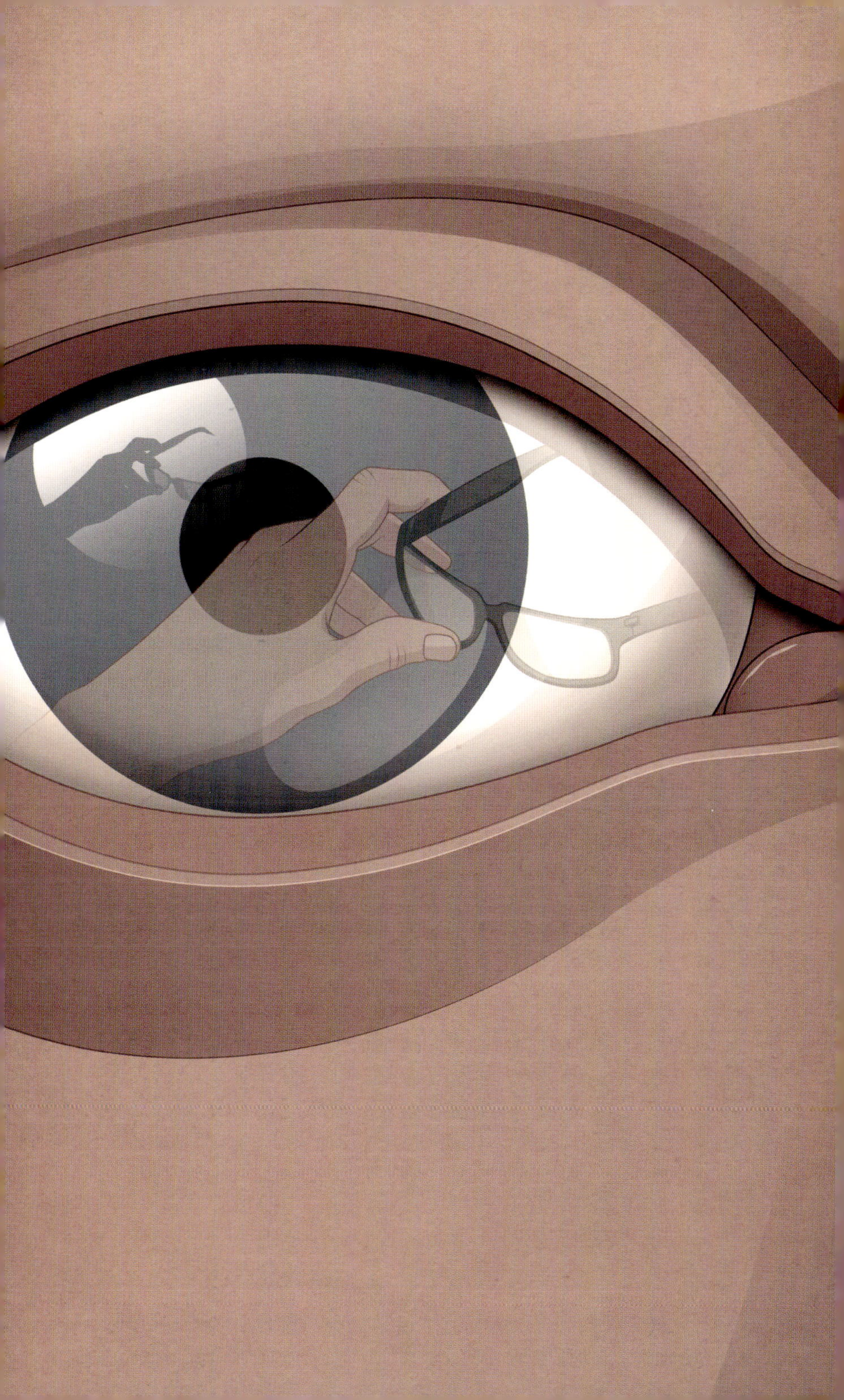

G.S

DR TSUTOMU SATO

In the 1930s Tsutomu Sato, a Japanese ophthalmologist, made the world's first attempt at vision correction surgery. Short-sightedness was recognised as being a major problem in the Japanese community. His technique was to make a series of very precise radial cuts (like the spokes of a bicycle wheel) on the inside surface of the cornea (see image page 88). Even then Sato recognised that the cornea – the front surface of the eye – was the key and that a surgeon needed to change its shape if he was going to repair the patient's short-sightedness.

> *"The great creators – the thinkers, the artists, the scientists, the inventors – stood alone against the men of their time. Every great new thought was opposed. Every great new invention was denounced. The first motor was considered foolish. The airplane was considered impossible. The power loom was considered vicious. Anaesthesia was considered sinful. But the men of unborrowed vision went ahead. They fought, they suffered and they paid. But they won."*
>
> ***Ayn Rand***

Sato's procedure was very successful at first, but within a year or so, disaster struck. His work predated medical knowledge of the importance of the inside layer of the cornea. It subsequently became apparent – partly through his work – that the inside layer of the cornea was critical to the health of the eye. The cornea is a series of layers. The front layer (or epithelium) can be scraped off as it reproduces itself all the time. However, the **back** layer (or endothelium) is similar to your brain cells in the sense that you are born with only a certain number. As you go through life you lose a few of these special cells, but they don't reproduce themselves. This back layer of the cornea has a critical role in keeping the cornea clear. It is where the cornea's fluid pump is located. Fluid is constantly being pumped out of the cornea by the cells in this back layer. If it is not pumping properly, your cornea becomes thick and waterlogged and your vision becomes cloudy, resulting in the need for a corneal transplant. The vital role of the back layer of the cornea was discovered partly through Sato's work but only became properly understood in the 1940s and 50s. We now know these things, whereas in the 1930s Dr Sato had no idea of the critical importance of the back layer of the cornea.

Dr Sato made incisions on the inside of the cornea with a blade and because it changed the shape of the cornea the procedure worked. He was hailed as a genius. Then, after about twelve months those cells that had been damaged ceased working properly and the cornea became swollen. Vision was lost and all of Dr Sato's patients needed to have corneal transplants.

Poor Dr Sato was devastated. He had, with the very best motives, initiated a ground-breaking procedure and for a short period of time it looked like he had found a solution to one of nature's oldest problems. Instead, he had created a nightmare for his patients and his fall from grace was so spectacular that for generations Japanese surgeons would not go anywhere near vision correction surgery. The shame that Sato had brought on himself and his profession was total. Even decades later Japanese ophthalmologists seemed to be almost unable to mention his name.

It wasn't until almost fifty years later that another ophthalmologist, the eccentric Russian genius, Svyatoslav Fyodorov, created history by successfully performing vision correction surgery by making radial cuts on the **front** of the cornea without any of Sato's horrible complications. After many long years in the professional wilderness, Dr Sato was recognised for his work in vision correction surgery. Like so many pioneers, he was thinking along the right lines, but was ahead of his time. ●

M.L

THE FEMTOSECOND LASER

If we want things to stay as they are, things will have to change.
Giuseppe di Lampedusa, Italian writer

Perhaps the most exciting development in ophthalmology in recent times has been the introduction of an amazing device with the hard-to-pronounce name, the *femtosecond laser*. Ten years ago about 95% of the vision correction procedures we carried out were done on the cornea (front surface of your eye) and only 5% of people had lens surgery (on the natural lens within your eye). In the last decade there has been a significant shift in these ratios and a much greater proportion of our patients are now having lens surgery than before.

Why has this happened? Well, for several reasons. Part of it is demographic – the bulk of our population are growing older. That big sector we call the baby boomers (those born between 1946 and 1964) are now in their 50s and 60s. They are, on the whole, a demanding group of people with a reasonable disposable income to whom life-style is important. I'm one of them, so I know! We don't want to be carting reading glasses around with us all the time, and also, let's be honest; we don't want to look 'old'. The baby boomers have driven a keen interest in vision correction by surgical means. They are our typical patients now where as ten years ago it was mainly younger, short-sighted people wanting to get rid of their distance glasses.

The second reason for the shift is the availability of much better artificial lenses to place inside your eye during lens surgery. These tiny intraocular lenses, designed to be placed inside your lens capsule, are just getting better and better. At the time they were first used, soon after World War II in England, they were just a little piece of hard plastic with the ability to give clear vision at one distance. Now you can get lenses that are specifically designed to deal with astigmatism, to deal with the error of long-sightedness or short-sightedness, and also to have a multifocal capacity so that you can keep both eyes pretty much the same and you can see in the distance and you can read.

But the major catalyst for this drift from cornea to lens surgery has been the introduction of the fantastic **femtosecond laser**.

What is a femtosecond?

Just to put you in the picture a *femto*second is a unit of time equal to 10^{-15} seconds. Let's get that into perspective: there are one thousand *milli*seconds in one second. There are *one million micro*seconds in one second ... and there are *one quadrillion* (or one million billion) *femto*seconds in one second.

One second is ...	*One thousand (10^3) milliseconds*
	One million (10^6) microseconds
	One billion (10^9) nanoseconds
	One trillion (10^{12}) picoseconds
	One quadrillion (10^{15}) femtoseconds

Most people know about *micro*seconds from watching Olympics' records tumble. They've never even heard of *femto*seconds! For context, ***a femtosecond is to a second what a second is to about 31.7 million years***. Right, so it's very fast. What does that actually mean?

How does the femtosecond laser work?

When a laser pulses at that speed, it is capable of dividing the targeted tissue at the molecular level and yet incredibly causes no heating or damage to the surrounding tissue. Instead of cutting, it actually breaks the molecular bonds that hold the tissue tightly together. We can now separate tissue without even touching your eye (apart from the suction ring, which holds the eye steady). Every pulse of the femtosecond laser creates a tiny expanding bubble of gas wherever it is targeted. These bubbles then all join up to create a space.

The Femtosecond laser and LASIK

In 2001 the femtosecond laser was used to create the flap in the first step of the LASIK procedure. The laser created a series of overlapping spaces just beneath the surface of the cornea. This allowed a flap of tissue to be freed from the underlying cornea.

Chris Rogers, Gerard Sutton and I introduced the femtosecond laser to Australia in October 2004 and the all-laser LASIK procedure became a reality.

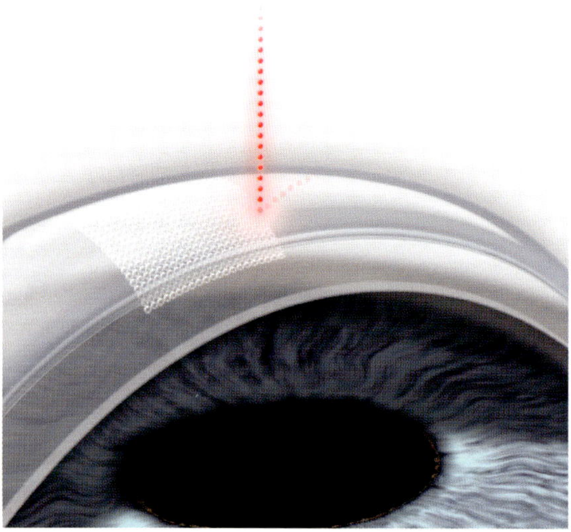

The femtosecond laser revolutionised the way the corneal flap was created for the first step in the LASIK procedure (see *LASIK*, page 57). As doctors, we had closely followed the success of the femtosecond laser in the US and had one waiting at the docks for delivery to our practice the day the TGA (Therapeutic Goods Administration) approved it for use in Australia. The femtosecond laser replaced the micro-keratome, an oscillating metal blade that was previously used to create the flap in LASIK. It was a huge leap forward for laser eye surgery. Here we had an instrument that could create this tiny flap of tissue without a blade ever touching the eye.

Overnight the femtosecond laser made LASIK safer, more accurate and more predictable than before. It has also been clinically shown to result in better vision for the patient. [4]

The Femtosecond laser and lens replacement surgery

Since then the femtosecond laser has been used to eliminate three of the manual steps of lens replacement surgery (see *Laser Lens Surgery*, page 90). Several of these manual steps that were done by hand or with an instrument are now done with the precision and reproducibility of the femtosecond laser. You can have your natural lens replaced if you have a cataract or, increasingly, as a vision correction procedure. Rather than changing your cornea we change your lens. This may be because your cornea is not suitable for laser vision correction. Or it may be because you are in an age group where cataract is going to affect you sooner or later; it makes more sense to replace your own natural lens even though it is not yet cloudy. As a result our vision correction plans often involve your lens, more so than previously.

The Femtosecond laser and SMILE

The femtosecond laser continued to inspire new techniques in vision correction surgery and in 2008 a new technique for reshaping the cornea was born. In femtosecond lenticule extraction, a thin, lens-shaped disc (or lenticule) was separated from the surrounding corneal tissue and then removed, resulting in the corneal shape required for clear unaided vision. This meant no corneal flap and no excimer laser. The procedure has further evolved to become SMILE laser, an acronym for small incision lenticule extraction. As the name suggests, the lenticule could now be extracted through a tiny laser-created keyhole incision in the cornea. SMILE was first introduced to Australia in 2012 and has found its place as a safe, accurate, and more modern procedure for correcting shortsightedness and astigmatism in many patients. The absence of a corneal flap means a less invasive procedure and less impact on corneal enervation compared to previous procedures. It is now emerging in the clinical data that SMILE laser may be a better choice for higher errors and drier eyes. ●

M.L

HOW FEMTOSECOND LASER LENS SURGERY CAME TO AUSTRALIA

How my colleagues and I were able to start performing femtosecond laser cataract surgery in Australia in April 2011 is an interesting story. Although it was obviously necessary to have a track record of credibility within the profession, there was also an element of luck to it in that I happened to be in the right place at the right time and became the first Australian to perform this new cataract procedure.

Everyone knew this was coming. The concept of the laser cataract work station had been talked about since 2005 and there were three different groups of international researchers developing the procedure. I knew and liked many of the people involved, but I had most faith in the Research and Development team from IntraLase because they had a few years earlier developed the IntraLase laser for LASIK. This same R&D team now worked for a new company called LenSx (subsequently owned by Alcon) and were involved in developing a femtosecond laser for cataract surgery.

In October 2010 I travelled to Chicago to attend a meeting of the American Academy of Ophthalmology where I caught up with Professor Michael Knorz, a German ophthalmologist whom I knew well, and Trudy Larkins, who at that stage was working for LenSx – the femtosecond laser company. I had been hoping to speak about the new laser cataract procedure at the Asia Pacific Academy of Ophthalmology which was meeting in Sydney in March 2011. At that stage there were only two femtosecond laser lens systems in operation anywhere in the world – one in Houston and another in Budapest. After discussing this with Professor Knorz, he pointed out that there was not enough time to get a laser cataract system set up in Sydney before the meeting. "Why don't we get a film crew together and ask Dr Zoltan Nagy if you can go to Budapest so that you could perform your first laser cataract procedure there?" Professor Knorz suggested.

It was a great idea, but one with loads of logistical problems. Later that night I emailed a senior executive at Alcon, who liked the idea and flicked it to Roy Acosta, the head of Alcon Asia Pacific. Roy is a larger than life, ex-USA army officer with the 101st Airborne, with a reputation for making the impossible happen. My proposal presented Roy with a dilemma. There is always intense competition in any industry to be the "first" to perform a new procedure, and ophthalmology is the same. There would have been over twenty practices vying for the honour of having one of their ophthalmologists perform the first laser cataract procedure in the region, and Roy Acosta would have to decide who that would be. This was where the reputation of Vision Eye Institute came into play. We had a long track record of embracing new technology and our professional standing was second to none. Also, VEI's ophthalmologists consistently reported on their experiences with new technology in a way that was of value to all cataract surgeons. In the end, Roy Acosta gave us the nod, and made it happen.

By February 2011 I found myself in a freezing Budapest surrounded by a film crew and a host of support people while I performed my first laser cataract procedure. Professor Zoltan Nagy generously allowed us to use his laser and also spent a lot of time training me in the finer points of how the laser altered the procedure. Even though I felt thoroughly prepared it was still incredibly nerve-racking. These were real patients. They spoke Hungarian and I spoke English, it was an unfamiliar operating environment, and it was all going to be captured on film. Thankfully, it all went perfectly and the film of that operation was shown at the APAO meeting in Sydney in March 2011. About a month after that we had our own system installed at Vision Eye Institute, in Sydney. That film became very popular around the world. It has been translated into Korean and Hindi, and somehow I have somehow ended up a minor celebrity in South Korea and India because of it.

All of this happened because of the encouragement and faith of our executives and partners at Vision Eye Institute, the R & D and marketing teams at Alcon and LenSx, and Professor Nagy in Budapest. They allowed us to play a role in opening up this technology to the world. ●

G.S

DR HAROLD RIDLEY

During the 1930s German chemists put acrylic acids through a polymerisation process to create a new material which they patented under the brand name 'Plexiglass' or Perspex.

Unlike glass, Perspex was easier to handle and more impact resistant. During World War 2 Perspex was introduced for such things as aircraft canopies and gun turrets. When machine gun bullets smashed into the canopy, the Perspex shattered on impact and pilots tended to suffer injuries to their eyes from flying shards of Perspex.

Nicholas Harold Lloyd Ridley was an ophthalmologist at Moorfields Hospital in London who began to see RAF fighter pilots with eye injuries caused by splinters of acrylic plastic or Perspex. What had an impact on Ridley was that none of the wounded pilots he examined who had pieces of Perspex in their eyes suffered adversely. When Perspex was lodged in the eye it did not trigger inflammation, which was what happened when patients had shards of glass in their eyes. Ridley concluded that it would be possible to make an artificial lens out of Perspex, which could then be inserted into the eye to correct cases of cataract. This concept was a breakthrough because up until that time the only option available for patients was to take the cataract out, surgically removing their entire lens. This invariably resulted in the patient suffering a very significant loss of focus and having to wear thick glasses afterwards.

Dr Ridley began developing and experimenting with a Perspex lens, which he could implant inside the eye to correct cases of cataract. On 29th November 1949 Ridley carried out the first implant of an intraocular lens. He pioneered this work despite there being staunch opposition from the medical community. Despite proceeding with his work in a careful and methodical manner, Ridley was pilloried by his peers. And whilst it is true that the procedure wasn't always successful – some of the lenses moved within the eye – the principle was sound. When a surgeon took out a cataract, it had to be replaced with something. During the 1950s and 1960s Ridley refined his technique and the quality of the Perspex lens improved. Slowly he gained acceptance for the procedure and today you would wonder what all the fuss was about. However, it is worth noting that the Food and Drug Administration in the US only approved the use of the intraocular lens as being "safe and effective" in 1981. Cataract extraction surgery with intraocular lens implantation is now the most common form of eye surgery in the world.

> *To see things in the seed,*
> *that is genius...*
> ***Lao Tzu***

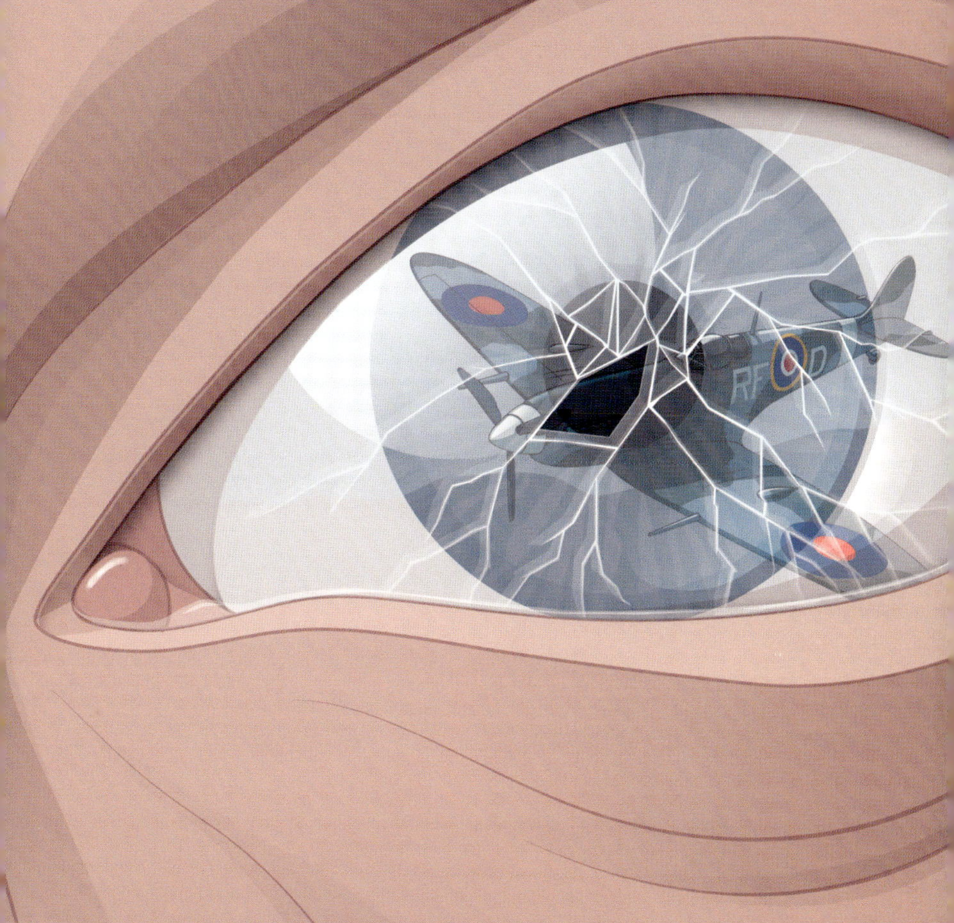

Today, Ridley is recognised as the father of modern cataract and lens surgery. He outlived almost two generations of his peers who opposed his work and was knighted by the Queen for his outstanding contribution to ophthalmology. ●

LASIK, ASLA AND SMILE LASER

There are three distinctly different corneal vision correction procedures available, ***LASIK***, ***PRK*** (known as ***ASLA*** at our practice) and ***SMILE*** laser. All three involve reshaping the cornea or front surface of your eye to the ideal shape to allow you to focus clearly without glasses.

Advanced Surface Laser – or **ASLA** – was first introduced to Australia by Peter Cohen, Chris Rogers and Michael Lawless in 1991, and involves reshaping the corneal surface with a cool, ultra-violet excimer laser. ASLA is still widely used but has been largely overshadowed by **LASIK**, which involves the creation of a microscopic flap in the cornea to allow the reshaping to occur *away from* the surface of the eye. By bypassing the ultra-sensitive surface of the eye, this results in far less discomfort during healing and a rapid visual recovery.

In both the LASIK and ASLA procedures, an excimer laser, in a matter of seconds, precisely removes a tiny quantity of tissue from your cornea. If you are short-sighted, the laser flattens your cornea by removing tissue from the centre. If you are long-sighted the laser makes your cornea more curved by removing tissue from the periphery. If you have astigmatism, the laser removes more tissue from some parts of the cornea than others, thus smoothing out the surface to a more regular shape. The laser is carefully programmed with the information it needs to treat your individual eye and remains within the doctor's control at all times. Due to the tiny involuntary movements of the eye, a special tracker 'locks on' to your eye and follows it at incredible speed to ensure that the laser treatment is delivered to precisely the right location on your cornea.

The third procedure, **SMILE laser**, removes the corneal tissue in an entirely different way. Instead of vaporising the tissue away, a very fast laser is used to separate a disc-shaped piece of your cornea from its surrounding tissue and this disc – or lenticule – is then removed from your cornea through a tiny laser-created keyhole incision. There is no corneal flap and there is no excimer laser involved. To date it is only suitable for short-sighted eyes (with or without astigmatism), but treatments for long-sightedness are expected to be available soon.

Read on for more detail about each of these fascinating procedures.

SMILE

Small incision lenticular extraction (or SMILE laser) is the latest application of the femtosecond laser. This incredibly fast laser was first used to create the flap in LASIK and subsequently to replace several of the manual steps in laser cataract surgery. Its most recent application in the world of vision correction surgery is in the SMILE laser procedure. In a single step the laser separates a thin, lens- shaped disc of tissue (a lenticule) from within the cornea. (*Fig. 1*, below).

Fig. 1

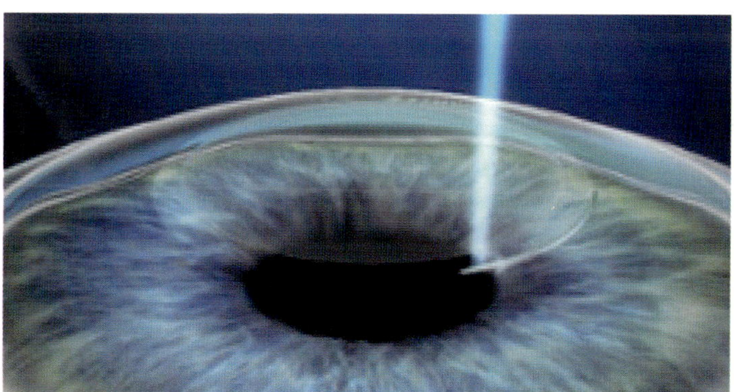

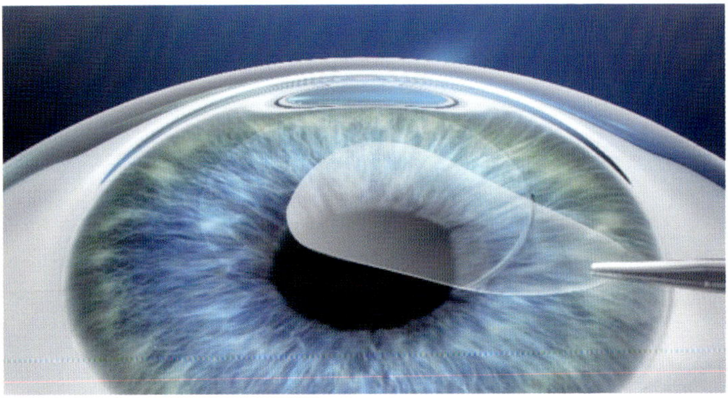

Fig. 2

This piece of tissue is then extracted through a tiny keyhole incision (*Fig. 2*, above), leaving the cornea with a new shape, enabling it to see clearly without glasses.

SMILE differs from LASIK in several ways: There is no tissue vaporised away in the SMILE laser procedure. The excimer laser – so essential to LASIK and ASLA – is not required. Instead of removing tissue by vaporising it, the unwanted tissue is simply separated from the rest and removed.

You can think about the excimer laser in LASIK and ASLA as being a little like a sander – reshaping the cornea by removing tissue one molecule at a time until the desired shape is achieved. The SMILE laser operates more like a bladeless lathe – defining a slice of corneal tissue which is then removed intact. The net effect on vision is exactly the same; whether you have LASIK, ASLA or SMILE, your cornea will take on a new shape which allows you to see clearly with the naked eye.

CASE STUDY

Rachel is 39 when she first comes to see me – about three years ago – to discuss vision correction surgery. She's a busy mother of three young kids and also works part-time as a pharmacist. She has been thinking about laser eye surgery for the past ten years but has been nervous about having it done – especially about any possible pain associated with the surgery or the recovery. Rachel is short-sighted – about –6 in each eye – and wears glasses most of the time. She used to wear contact lenses but has found them increasingly uncomfortable over the past few years. She suffers from a dry eye condition which means she has to use artificial tears several times a day. She sees a dry eye specialist who has dramatically improved her ocular surface but she has to work hard to stay on top of it.

Rachel has the battery of tests we put all our patients through and I can see that she has nice thick corneas, with plenty of tissue available to treat her -6 prescription. But I am reluctant to offer LASIK to Rachel because of her dry eye condition. LASIK involves the creation of a thin flap of corneal tissue which is folded out of the way while the laser reshapes the underlying tissue. The flap is then replaced and heals very quickly, resulting in almost instant visual recovery and very little discomfort. However, the creation of the flap causes a temporary reduction in the amount of reflex tears secreted into the eyes. We have a tear gland above each eye that constantly releases watery (aqueous) tears into the eye in response to feedback from the eye's surface. If you cut an onion, for example, the eye's surface is irritated and a lot more reflex tears are released into the eye to flush it out and soothe it. The nerves which stimulate these reflex tears are situated in the surface of the cornea and they are temporarily affected by creating the flap in LASIK. The result is that less reflex tears are produced – especially in the first few weeks after LASIK. This is why all LASIK patients are given artificial tears to use liberally for the first few weeks after a LASIK procedure.

Rachel has the battery of tests we put all our patients through and I can see that she has nice thick corneas, with plenty of tissue available to treat her -6 prescription. But I am reluctant to offer LASIK to Rachel because of her dry eye condition.

But for some people, especially if they already have an underlying dry eye condition, the temporary dryness becomes more long term and can really take the good out of having a great result from LASIK. Their eyes may not actually feel any drier – because they have reduced sensation – but their vision can be affected and fluctuate depending on the hydration state of their eyes. In our experience, people with underlying dry eye that persists even when treated, tend to have these lingering issues after LASIK and it is one of the common reasons we would steer clear of LASIK and recommend a surface procedure (ASLA) instead. ASLA gives the same results as LASIK and the procedure itself is quick and painless, but ASLA has a much slower visual recovery and much more discomfort during healing. Until recently, ASLA accounted for about 10% of our corneal vision correction patients, while LASIK accounted for 90%.

The great thing about SMILE is that the procedure is performed deeper in the cornea than LASIK – which reshapes the superficial layers directly beneath the microscopic flap. The SMILE laser procedure preserves the corneal nerves intact and this means far less impact on dry eye patients.

I explained to Rachel that LASIK would likely aggravate her dry eye and that ASLA was a much better option for her. But she didn't want to have ASLA. With her busy schedule she just couldn't afford the down-time of a week or two where she may not able to drive or read fine detail at work. She was also terrified of any pain or discomfort – which ASLA would almost certainly cause for a couple of days. (Incidentally, this discomfort is managed with oral medications, topical drops and the use of a contact lens that acts like a bandage, and is rarely an issue for most people).

Rachel decided to stick with glasses for the time being and perhaps return when she was a bit older and have a lens replacement instead.

Then along came SMILE laser... We installed the latest laser vision correction technology in late 2014 and now recommend SMILE laser as one option for all suitable candidates. It reshapes the cornea by defining and separating a disc of tissue within the cornea, which is removed through a keyhole incision. So far it is suitable for prescription ranges from about -3 up to -10 (including any astigmatism). The great thing about SMILE is that the procedure is performed deeper in the cornea than LASIK – which reshapes the superficial layers directly beneath the microscopic flap. The SMILE laser procedure preserves the corneal nerves intact and this means far less impact on dry eye patients. Studies are now starting to show that SMILE laser may give a better result than LASIK for those with higher errors.

Sure enough, within about a month of the installation of our new SMILE laser, Rachel was back! She had followed the news on our website and noted with interest the advent of the SMILE technique. Her eyes were much the same as before, only this time we could offer her a procedure that wouldn't aggravate her dry eye. She had both eyes treated with the SMILE procedure and within a couple of days (and no discomfort) later, she could see with crisp 20-20 vision – without glasses or contacts. To Rachel it was well worth waiting for; she can do more with her kids and enjoy life to the full without her heavy glasses. And she hardly missed a beat. She had surgery on a Friday and was back at work the following week. Now there's something to SMILE about!

LASIK

All around the world, the majority of all patients undergoing vision correction surgery still have LASIK. That stands for **LAS**er **I**n-situ **K**eratomileusis. The **laser** in question is the excimer laser used to remodel the cornea (under the flap) during the procedure in order to create a corneal shape that will focus light clearly without glasses or contact lenses. **I**n-situ means that the procedure is carried out on live, intact corneal tissue in its original position (as distinct from tissue that has been removed from the cornea). **K**eratomileusis comes from 'kerato', which is a Greek-derived prefix meaning cornea, and 'mileusis', which means to remodel, or reshape.

Fig 1.

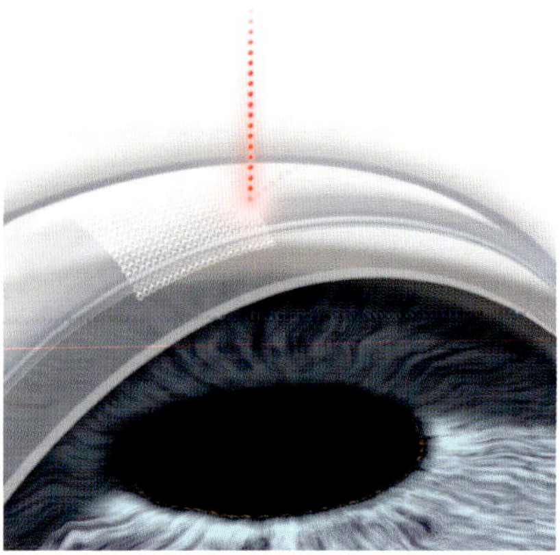

First, a special laser called a femtosecond laser (*see page 44*) creates a thin flap of tissue (one tenth of a millimeter in thickness) on the surface of your cornea. This flap is created without a blade ever touching your eye (*Fig 1*).

Then the flap is carefully folded back to reveal the underlying corneal stroma (*Fig 2*).

Next, a cool ultraviolet laser called an excimer laser reshapes the underlying tissue to the required shape for clear vision without glasses or contact lenses (*Fig 3*).

Fig 2.

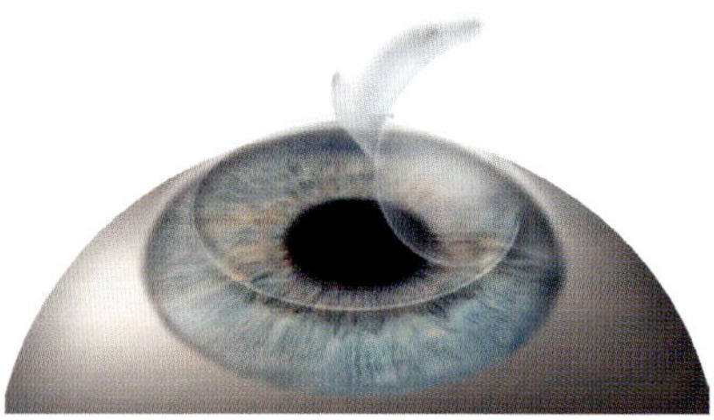

Then the flap of corneal tissue is very carefully replaced.

LASIK was first introduced to Australia in 1995. Unlike the previously dominant ASLA (PRK) procedure, LASIK allows us to bypass the tear film and the surface layers of the cornea. Because of this, the usual inflammation process that kicks in after ASLA does not occur with LASIK. The eye stays quiet and white and comfortable. The huge advantage of LASIK over ASLA is that you have almost instant visual recovery and you have almost no discomfort.

Fig 3.

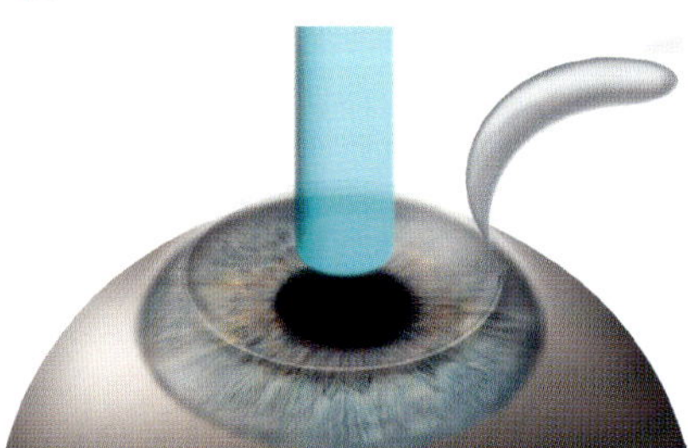

CASE STUDY

Here's a typical scenario: Jason comes to see me. He's the husband of one of my staff and has only come in reluctantly as

Flap, Zap and Put it Back

LASIK still remains the most common refractive surgical procedure in the world, even though it has recently lost some ground to the newer SMILE laser procedure. LASIK involves the creation of a corneal flap one tenth of a millimetre in thickness with a femtosecond laser, the re-shaping of the underlying cornea with an excimer laser and then the replacement of the flap.

I hesitate to quote the oft used short-hand for the technique; "Flap, Zap and put it back". This phrase certainly captures the basic surgical steps but belittles the sophisticated nuances of the surgery and makes it sound both perfectly simple and perfectly safe. While I would argue that LASIK is a safe procedure – I've had it done, myself – I would also assert that no vision correction procedure is either perfectly safe or perfectly predictable. However, what has been firmly established is that LASIK is very accurate, (especially for low to moderate levels of short-sightedness) and the visual recovery is rapid.

he is not keen on the idea of laser eye surgery but is now desperate to get away from his reading glasses. He's your typical under-the-pump, corporate type with two little kids – we all know the story. Jason is forty-four years old and has in the past had pretty good all-round vision. However, since the age of about forty, he has needed reading glasses for small print. No problems so far. Increasingly however, he needs to use these glasses for more and more visual tasks. From what he tells me I suspect he's starting to drive his wife up the wall because he can't see things he should be able to see. He can't see the head of a screw to tell if he needs a flat-head or Phillips-head screwdriver to loosen it. When it's his turn to give the baby her medicine in the middle of the night he can't see what dose of Panadol he's measuring out. Now, he has to cart his glasses everywhere with him but keeps losing them. Jason's distance sight is still pretty good and he's not interested in wearing glasses full-time.

When I examine his eyes, it is clear that he is ideal for LASIK. Nice thick corneas, a low prescription (he is long-sighted, about +1 for distance and a bit more for near, same in both eyes), nice healthy eyes. His right eye is his dominant eye. That means the one he favours or relies on more. This eye is providing more regular feedback to his visual cortex, that part of the brain that interprets what we see, than the other eye. Because Jason is forty-four years old we need to factor presbyopia into his vision correction plan. He will need a form of blended vision to maximise his independence from glasses. And so I advise him that, subject to a successful contact lens trial to 'test-drive' the final result, we can go ahead and do a LASIK procedure on his eyes. He will need LASIK on both eyes because, although he can see quite well in the distance, that is only through using his natural lens's focusing power to the maximum and that will change over the next few years so that his distance will also start to become blurry.

Surprisingly, he's not keen on the contact lens trial at all and has a pretty bad phobia about anyone touching his eyes. This happens! Some people just get all weird about anyone coming near their eyes. We are used to it and the staff optometrists are very well trained at dealing with it so before he knows it he is happily wearing a pair of 'trial' contact lenses for the day to see how he gets on. His wife takes them out for him that evening and he declares the trial a complete success – he could see everything he needed to see and his vision for driving still felt normal and comfortable. So, he was scheduled for LASIK to both eyes. We target his right eye to be perfectly clear for distance and his left eye to be a little less clear for distance but a bit clearer for reading. This is the blended vision effect. And despite being a very nervous patient – he definitely needed the Valium we routinely offer all our laser vision correction patients – he was absolutely delighted with his out-come the next morning.

Surprisingly, he's not keen on the contact lens trial at all and has a pretty bad phobia about anyone touching his eyes. This happens! Some people just get all weird about anyone coming near their eyes.

He remarked on the sense of freedom he immediately felt, not having to carry his reading glasses everywhere with him. (See page 73 for Jason's first-hand account of his LASIK procedure.)

There have been some major advancements in the LASIK procedure in the past ten years. Now that we are using the femtosecond laser to create the flap there is less manual intervention by the surgeon. The entire procedure is under the doctor's control, but there is less manual involvement than there was before 2004 when we were using the microkeratome. It is more precise in the way that the flap is created with the laser. There is no way that the blade could achieve the same effect in the same predictable fashion.

Also the way that the laser tracks the eye has improved. The eye is moving all the time. It is constantly making tiny movements that we are not even aware of so that we are able to see without having to move (see *A Remarkable Instrument*, page 18). You can see stationary objects even when your eyes appear to be still because your eyes are making tiny movements all the time, and those movements would affect the result of the laser surgery if they weren't compensated for. The eye is tracked during the LASIK procedure by a highly specialised tracking device. It is actually based on the NASA technology used in missile tracking devices. The tracker locks onto the eye and any movement that the eye makes is mirrored. The laser repositions itself thousands of times per second to track the eye and ensure the laser energy is delivered to the exact location it is targeted to.

LASIK is not a one-size-fits-all procedure though, as the following case studies show:

CASE STUDY

Sharon came to see me for a vision correction consultation about two years ago. She was quite short-sighted (-8) and heavily dependent on glasses and her soft contact lenses, which she wore most of the time. Sharon worked in marketing full-time and had three young kids. She was ready to make a break with contact lenses and take the plunge. Financially, she explained to me, it was costing her a small fortune to wear daily disposable contact lenses as well as keep a nice pair of glasses and prescription sunglasses. She was planning on financing her laser eye surgery over two years to spread out the cost. One of the first tests that we do during the initial consultation is a special topographical map of the cornea. It's called an Orbscan. It tells us a lot, not only about the thickness of the cornea but also about its shape.

The average cornea is about half a millimetre thick (0.5mm or 500 microns). Sharon's corneas were only 470 microns in thickness, which is thinner than average. Coupled with that she had a high prescription (-8) and, to make things worse, her cornea wasn't just thin, it was also a very steep shape in the centre. This makes it more vulnerable to ectasia after laser eye surgery, a rare complication where the cornea becomes weak and unstable. So, despite her keenness to proceed, I had to break the news to her that a corneal procedure would just not be appropriate for her.

Perhaps in five or six years' time, as she approaches her fifties, we could look at doing a lens replacement procedure for her. At the moment though, her own natural lens is giving her the huge advantage of being able to change her focus from distance to near. So, no vision correction procedure for Sharon for the time being.

Victoria's story starts off very similar to Sharon's. Victoria came to see me for an initial consultation about a year ago. She was also short-sighted (-8) just like Sharon, in her late thirties and growing tired of glasses. The thing that bothered her most about her short-sightedness was that she had to get so close to the mirror to put on her eye make-up that she invariably ended up with mascara on the mirror ...! Her corneal maps showed beautifully thick, regularly-shaped corneas with plenty of tissue to spare, even with her relatively high glasses prescription. Victoria was an extremely cautious person when it came to her eyes. She had researched laser eye surgery for years and finally taken her GP's advice to come and see me for a consultation about her unique case. The problem with online research is that it tells you nothing about your own particular eyes. I had a long discussion with Victoria on the type of procedure that would give her the best outcome – which was LASIK. She actually saw another ophthalmologist for a second opinion before going ahead with her surgery with me. She just wanted to be sure that she had all the relevant information. Her procedure was very straight-forward. And, apart from being able to apply her mascara in comfort now, Victoria's favourite thing about her new eyes is that she can wear designer sunglasses for the first time! ●

The problem with online research is that it tells you nothing about your own particular eyes.

G.S

WHAT DO THE LATEST STUDIES ON LASIK SHOW?

A recent study highlights that 96 per cent of pilots in active service for the US Armed Forces reported that their visual acuity improved after LASIK surgery. These people have the highest visual acuity needs of any individual. There couldn't be a more stringent test.

For naval pilots within a defence group – those who fly ultra-fast planes and land them on aircraft carriers in challenging weather conditions in countries involved in war – good vision is clearly a matter of life or death.

Understandably then, in past decades, many highly competent young men and women, intent on pursuing a career in the armed services, have been turned away, just because their vision has let them down.

Fortunately, times have changed and so have the advances in vision correction surgery. These advances have enabled talented individuals to pursue their dreams in the armed services with more precise vision than they could ever have imagined.

In America, armed forces personnel are able to undergo free vision correction surgery on a priority basis as part of the Warfighter Refractive Eye Surgery Programme (WRESP).

WRESP is a significant medical program which was started after numerous large studies were completed to assess the impact of vision correction surgery on actively deployed military personnel. The US armed forces' two preferred methods of vision correction surgery are ASLA (also referred to as PRK) and LASIK.

One clinical study that has come out of the program looked at the outcomes of LASIK on naval aviators – an occupation, I would argue, that has amongst the highest visual needs of any.

Specifically, the study looked at visual outcomes, safety and quality of vision following LASIK. It was carried out at two naval sites and included over 600 eyes, (of which 548 were short-sighted). The findings were significant:

- **98%** of myopic (short-sighted) eyes achieved a 20/20 result.
- **40%** of short-sighted and astigmatic eyes were able to read at least one extra line of best corrected vision on the eye test chart compared to before surgery.
- **96%** of hyperopic (long-sighted) eyes achieved a 20/20 result.
- **95.6%** of pilots believed the surgery had helped their effectiveness as naval aviators
- A whopping **99.6%** would recommend it to their friends.

This study is significant in a number of ways. Firstly, if the US Navy thinks this surgery is safe for its aviators who fly multimillion dollar jets, then the irrational fear and fear-mongering about the safety of LASIK in appropriately screened patients should be put to rest. Secondly, the visual outcomes are excellent, and for appropriately selected patients, the most likely visual outcome is 20/20. [4]

Success brings disadvantages too. The success of the Warfighter programme has also come at a logistic price for the US armed forces. A New York Times article (June 2006) described a new problem for the US Navy arising from the improved vision of active and would-be pilots: "Aging fighter pilots can now remain in the cockpit longer, reducing annual recruiting needs. And recruits whose bad vision once would have disqualified them from the Special Forces are now eligible, making the competition for these coveted slots even tougher."

The author went on to state that as a result: "For generations, Academy graduates with high grades and bad eyes were funnelled into the submarine service. But in the five years since the Naval Academy began offering free eye surgery to all midshipmen, it has missed its annual quota for supplying the navy with submarine officers every year." ●

CASE STUDY: AN AUSTRALIAN PERSPECTIVE

Like many ophthalmologists in Australia, I provide a consulting and surgical service to our armed service personnel.

Vision correction surgery has been available to certain armed forces personnel in Australia for over a decade. Funding has been provided for those in specific roles such as SAS and Naval Divers. Strict screening and follow-up guidelines have been put in place to ensure optimal function prior to a return to active duty.

One of the patients I have worked with was a 39-year-old Australian naval pilot. The naval pilot was referred to our practice for assessment for vision correction surgery. He was flying helicopters and found that not only was his astigmatism causing distortion in his vision – which was disconcerting – he also found that his spectacles affected his peripheral vision. He was an active sportsman who enjoyed surfing and soccer.

The naval pilot had moderate astigmatism, but corrected to 20/20 in both eyes with his glasses on. I discussed with him the risks and benefits of the surgery and stressed the impact that any adverse event would have on his ability to fly helicopters. At this point in time pilots in the Royal Australian Airforce must have Advanced Surface Laser (ASLA) rather than LASIK (although this is a legacy from many years ago, when ASLA had at the time a lower complication rate than LASIK, which is no longer the case). Interestingly, pilots in the Australian Army and Navy can have LASIK or ASLA.

The Lieutenant proceeded to have a surface laser procedure to each eye and by three months, he had achieved uncorrected vision of 20/20 in each eye. He underwent his compulsory six-month review and was cleared to fly without glasses. He continues to fly helicopters for the Royal Australian Navy and enjoys his surfing and soccer without the need for glasses.

What puzzles me, as a true believer in vision correction surgery, is that despite improvements in corneal and lens vision correction techniques, the uptake remains very low.

Since LASIK was first introduced to Australia in 1995 only an estimated 2–3 per cent of the eligible population have taken up the surgical option. What are the reasons for such a low uptake? I imagine there are several reasons; contact lenses have continued to improve and for many people, spectacles are not only perfectly acceptable, they are a fashion accessory. Cost is also a barrier for many patients, especially in these uncertain economic conditions. Patients quite reasonably want some certainty surrounding their investment. However, for many people it is the fear of a catastrophic event that stops them from proceeding. In reality this risk for LASIK is extremely low but for many people, the fact that it is even a possibility is enough to deter them. We have never had an IntraLase LASIK disaster at our practice and the risk of a catastrophic result is believed to be 1 in 5,000 or less. It is also interesting to note that the risk of a sight-threatening complication from soft contact lens wear is in the order of 1 in 16,000 wearers per year.[5]

Hopefully, published studies such as the LASIK one conducted by the U.S. Armed Services will finally convince those eye care professionals who remain hesitant, and their patients, of the life-changing results that can be achieved from this most common of surgeries.

M.L

ASLA (Advanced Surface Laser)

When we first introduced the excimer laser to Australia back in 1991, all vision correction procedures were performed on the *surface* of the cornea. Back then we called it PRK (which stands for Photo Refractive Keratectomy) but as techniques improved it became known as Advanced Surface Laser (or ASLA). Although the majority of vision correction procedures we perform are now LASIK or SMILE laser, ASLA still plays an important role. One is not better than the other in terms of outcome or safety. They have different uses and suitability for different patients. When you perform laser vision correction on the surface of the eye you still use an excimer laser but it doesn't involve creating a flap as in LASIK.

It is a lot simpler for a surgeon to just operate on the surface of the eye compared to creating a flap. We still have to prepare the eye's surface by removing the epithelium and the tear film layers. During the procedure, those layers are disrupted with a solution of alcohol and removed, exposing the smooth regular surface of the cornea beneath. *(Fig 1)*

The next step involves using the excimer laser to reshape the cornea to the required shape for clear vision without glasses or contact lenses. *(Fig 2)*

You get beautiful results. It is a fantastic procedure and great for someone who has a thinner cornea, but there is definitely more discomfort during the healing process after the surgery. You can't see properly for the first few days after your procedure and it is usually a couple of weeks before you start to see clearly. It takes that length of time for your epithelium (front surface of your eye) to re-establish itself on the cornea and to build up to a nice smooth layer again.

Fig 1.

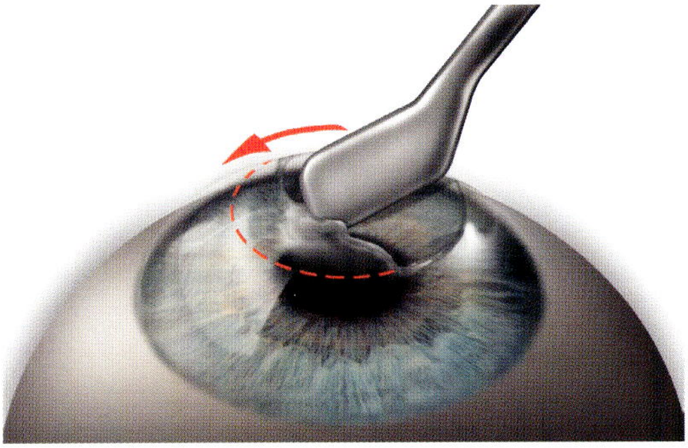

ASLA is certainly more comfortable than it was ten years ago because we use a bandage contact lens on the surface of the eye and we use Voltaren eye drops as well as pain relief medication. But you have to be prepared for a bit of discomfort. Some people describe it as very scratchy eyes. You feel like you have a grain of sand in

Fig 2.

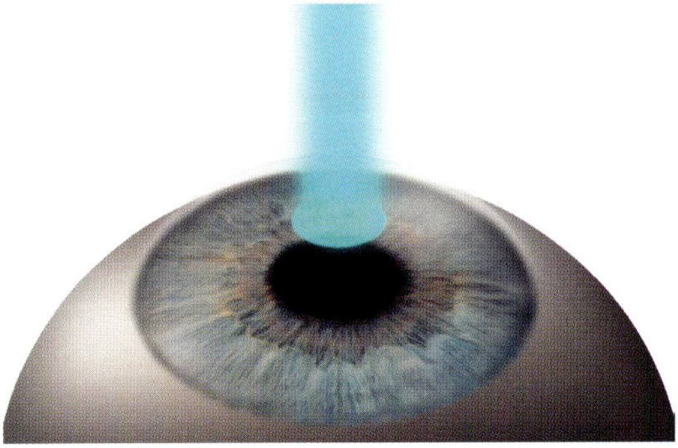

your eyes. It varies. One of the staff had it done and she has sinus problems and said it was nothing compared to her sinus problems. Other people say they can barely open their eyes. A lot of it depends on the individual's pain threshold and what else is going on in their lives. ASLA is certainly something you get done when you have a little bit of down time, whereas with LASIK or SMILE laser you go in and have it done then just go back to work within a day or two. (With LASIK you're advised to take the next day off but in most cases you don't really have to once you have had your post-operative visit and been given the thumbs-up by your surgeon. SMILE laser takes a couple of days to reach optimum vision).

With LASIK you typically have excellent vision the next morning. We check the vision the morning after your procedure and if you had LASIK you generally have 20/20 vision. With ASLA you would be struggling. But while there is quite a difference in the immediate result, there is no difference in the long term result.

While the majority of people are suitable for LASIK, ASLA may be the procedure of choice in certain circumstances, e.g. if your cornea is too thin for LASIK, has any unusual steepness, or in certain dry eye conditions (although SMILE laser is probably a better option for these dry eye patients, where it is available). Your doctor will choose the one that is suited to your eyes and that is going to give you the best result.

Of patients undergoing laser vision correction on the cornea at our practice, about 60-70% still have LASIK versus 15-20% each for ASLA and SMILE. Why does LASIK dominate? Because we use the femtosecond laser to create the flap, LASIK is a very predictable and accurate procedure. It caters for a wide range of spectacle prescriptions. And because you have little or no down-time, as well as instant visual recovery and generally no pain, it is the procedure of choice for the majority of people, assuming they are suitable to have a flap.

There are some reasons that preclude you from having LASIK – for example, having a thinner cornea. If you have a very thin cornea, ASLA (Advanced Surface Laser) comes into its own because you have all that extra tissue to work with that you would have allocated to a flap in LASIK. ASLA also has implications for people with ocular surface issues such as dry eye, so there are certain patients that are more suited to it as the following example illustrates:

CASE STUDY

Leanne is a classic example of an ASLA patient. She came to see us seeking that elusive quarry, freedom from eyewear. Having worn glasses since starting high school, Leanne was about -6 (short-sighted) and had a fairly stable prescription for the previous two years. At twenty-eight years of age she was a busy partner in a law firm in the city and also swam competitively. She told me that she was getting married soon, and wanted to get rid of her glasses 'forever'! At first, she looked like the perfect choice for LASIK. But, when we looked carefully at her eyes, things were not as straight-forward as they first appeared. For a start, she suffered from dry eye, which made contact lens wear very difficult for her. Her dry eye stemmed from her oily tear production. Our watery tears are produced in our lacrimal gland, tucked away above the eye. These are the tears that are stimulated by irritation to our eye (cutting an onion or getting something in your eye) as well as emotion (tears of sadness, joy and so on). This component of our tears consists mostly of water. They flush out and hydrate the eyes as well as provide a nice smooth, shiny surface on the cornea so we can see clearly. But these tears are no good on their own as they can easily evaporate if they are not protected by a layer of oily tears. The oily tears are produced in a little row of glands along the eyelids (upper and lower) and they continuously squeeze tiny amounts of oil into the tear layer. So here was one of the problems: Leanne's eyelids were not producing nice oily tears. They were

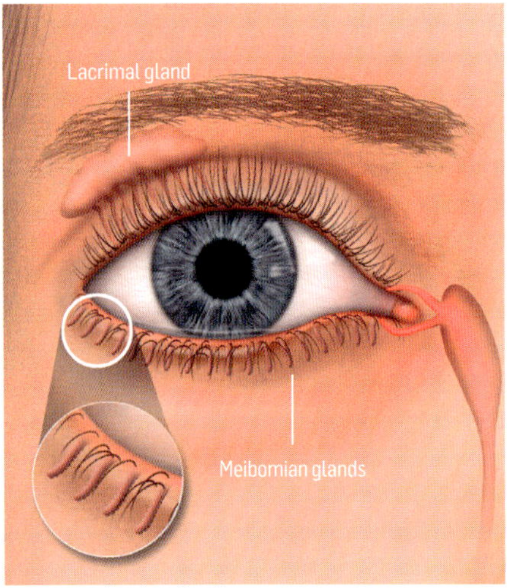

producing very little as most of the glands were blocked and if you did squeeze some out it was a thick white substance – like toothpaste in consistency - and not suitable for coating the watery tear layer. This condition is called meibomian gland dysfunction and it's pretty common.

The other issue with Leanne's eyes was that although her corneas looked healthy and normal they were thinner than average. Unfortunately, her corneas were not thick enough to allow me to treat all of her -6.0 prescription safely with LASIK. One of the possible risks with LASIK is corneal ectasia – a condition where the cornea becomes inherently weak after surgery because it is too thin. This is something we used to occasionally see many years ago, in the early days of LASIK. However, the limitations of LASIK are now well understood and part of the patient selection process is to ensure that the cornea is the right thickness and shape to successfully undergo LASIK.

Now, there were two issues to consider: the dry eye and the thin cornea. Both of these are reasons not to choose LASIK, or certainly to think very carefully about it. Leanne was pretty excited about having laser eye surgery and had requested LASIK because that was what her fiancé had recently had (and loved). So, I explained to her that as she had an abnormal tear film that we needed to address first. This would involve some lid hygiene (basically wiping the margins of her eyelashes every day with a special solution to dissolve away the deposits that were blocking her tear glands). Warm compresses would help speed things up. And lots of artificial tears would support her tear film while the glands recovered. Her problem was not particularly bad, but from experience we know that after LASIK there is always a bit of temporary dry eye and this can be a lot more of a nuisance if there is a pre-existing tear film issue. So it would have to be addressed first.

The second issue was that her cornea was too thin for LASIK so if she wanted to have a vision correction procedure she would instead need to have a surface laser procedure (ASLA). Although it would give an identical outcome to LASIK, it would involve a bit more down time. At which stage Leanne burst into tears! Nothing wrong with her lacrimal gland… She was just disappointed because she had set her expectations on her fiancé's experience. Several tissues and a cup of coffee later she calmed down enough to say she would think about it. And that's absolutely fine. The decision to have vision correction surgery should never be rushed. It takes time to digest all the things that have been explained to you, especially the issues that are unique to your particular eyes.

Whilst I like it that patients do their own independent research, I do caution them about trying to find out everything they need to know on Google. You could research vision correction surgery on Google until the cows come home but you will be no wiser as to what procedure is going to maximise your unique experience.

Whilst I like it that patients do their own independent research, I do caution them about trying to find out everything they need to know on Google. You could research vision correction surgery on Google until the cows come home but you will be no wiser as to what procedure is going to maximise your unique experience.

About three weeks later Leanne's optometrist called me to say that she had sought another opinion and was booked in to have LASIK at St Elsewhere, but she had suddenly lost her nerve and wanted to come and see us again…. What could I say? The poor girl was just so stressed out about the wedding and work and her eyes that she was almost a nervous wreck. I saw her and explained to her that I was offering her the best vision correction plan for her unique situation and that I was very confident that it was going to be a success or else I wouldn't have suggested it in the first place. This meant no LASIK surgery, but instead ASLA, a surface laser procedure. Leanne agreed and did the dry eye therapy – and there was a big improvement after only three or four weeks. Then we scheduled the ASLA procedure for her eyes on a Friday morning and she took the next week off work. Her vision had improved enough the following week for her to return to work and it slowly improved over the next two weeks. She came to see us about three weeks after her procedure and she had better than 20/20 vision in both eyes – in fact better vision than she had ever had with her glasses. She was a very happy girl and looked radiant in the wedding photo she sent us a couple of months later.

Dry eye can be a big concern when choosing a vision correction procedure. Some patients don't have Leanne's success in treating their dry eye, especially middle-aged women due to the hormonal effect on their tear production. This is often the reason that LASIK is not the procedure of choice for certain candidates for vision correction.

Since October 2014, we have been able to offer suitable patients a SMILE laser procedure instead of LASIK or ASLA. SMILE is minimally invasive on the cornea, causes less disruption to corneal nerve supply and may be a better option that LASIK for some dry eye patients.

Your LASIK, SMILE or ASLA procedure

So, what's it like to actually have a laser vision correction procedure like LASIK, ASLA or SMILE? I can tell you from my own experience that it is all over before you know it. It really is a very quick procedure. Jason (one of our earlier case studies) gives this account of the big event:

On the day of my LASIK procedure I was nervous. In fact I hadn't slept that well the night before. Rationally, I could tell myself over and over that it was a safe operation and that they wouldn't have recommended it for me if I wasn't a perfect candidate but I still felt nervous! My wife actually works at the laser eye surgery centre and, as an optometrist, has seen hundreds of successful cases of LASIK – the procedure I would be having – and has been encouraging me to have it for a while now.

My wife drops me off in the morning and the whole thing takes about two hours. Shortly after I arrive I am offered a Valium, which certainly takes the edge off the nerves and I start to feel quite positive about the whole thing.

The Laser Suite consists of a couple of highly-specialised rooms full of high-tech equipment and lots of busy-looking staff in scrubs – all very professional-looking.

The whole thing takes less than 30 seconds. There is a loud clicking noise and lots of flashing lights and then it is over.

It is my turn and the first step is to create the flaps on my corneas. I lie down on a special bed in the first room and my head is positioned under an expensive-looking machine - the femtosecond laser - that is about to create a flap in my cornea. The nurse puts a couple of eye drops into my eyes – to numb them she explains. Don't hold back on them, I think. Then they talk me through the process where the machine actually presses onto my eye for what seems like a very short time – 15 seconds, I later discover – and the same for the other eye and that is that bit out of the way! My vision is blurry and my heart is still beating very fast, even though there wasn't much sensation of anything apart from some pressure on my eyes and everything going dark momentarily.

Then I am lead into a larger, adjoining room. I lie on the operating table and the doctor talks to me about my procedure. I'm in the zone now and just nod and try to relax. The second part of the procedure is where the excimer laser actually reshapes my corneas to a new shape so I can see without glasses. The whole thing takes less than 30 seconds. There is a loud clicking noise and lots of flashing lights and then it is over. There is the sensation of cool liquid on my eye and after a short break they do the other eye. It doesn't hurt although there is some discomfort from the lid speculum, which is holding my eye open all the time. Apparently there is a tracking system in use on the laser, which follows the tiny movements of my eye, even as I try my best to look at the light. It locks onto the pattern of my iris and follows me around so the laser can do its job in exactly the right place.

Before I know it I am back in the waiting area again, with some clear eye shields taped to my eyes to protect them overnight while the flap heals. They will also prevent me from accidentally rubbing my eyes in my sleep. The eye drops leave my eyes feeling a bit sensitive to light and I realise that I am overcome with tiredness – partly from not having slept much last night and partly from the emotional toll it has taken on me. My wife drives me home and I rest for a while and my eyes feel a bit scratchy so I take the tablets they provided for me and I sleep a little.

When I wake up an hour or so later I peek out from behind my eye shields and am very excited to see that I can already read – even small print – without my glasses!

ASLA and SMILE laser are very similar in terms of the patient experience; preparation is identical but in both cases the procedure is quicker, as there is no corneal flap created.

It is interesting to hear our patients' different perspectives on the procedure. The acclaimed action thriller writer, Matthew Reilly, describes his LASIK procedure in his own inimitable style…

"When I went in for my laser procedure, I was quite surprised my head wasn't put in a vice or anything – I was just lying on a bed with a little indentation for my head. Someone said 'Stay still,' and I thought, 'damned right I'll stay still…' They whipped open a flap on my eyeball – went in – zapped the cornea – and put the flap back down again. Amazing stuff – it was over in minutes. Everything they said would happen did happen. That afternoon and evening my eyesight was a bit foggy– a bit like opening the doors of your car on a cold day when you fog up the windows – but when I woke up the next morning everything was crystal clear. It was all just so seamlessly done and the results speak for themselves. My eye-sight is better than 20/20 and I have become a sunglasses hoarder, now that I can buy whatever sunglasses I like." ●

The future – LASIK and ASLA vs SMILE laser

Up until very recently, LASIK reigned supreme; if you were short-sighted (with or without astigmatism) or if you were a little long-sighted (as long as your lenses were clear and corneas were suitable) LASIK was the first choice of vision correction procedure. Nothing could touch it in terms of accuracy, speed of recovery and safety.

But things are always evolving in the world of vision correction. Since its inception, doctors and researchers have worked tirelessly to improve the results – the vision, the accuracy and the safety profile. The introduction of the SMILE laser technique to Australia in 2012 has knocked LASIK off its perch to some degree. Granted, not many vision correction clinics offer SMILE at this stage – partly due to the very high set-up cost – but studies continue to show that SMILE laser offers some advantages over LASIK that cannot be overlooked: The SMILE procedure is performed deeper within the cornea, it has less impact on the strength of the cornea – that all-important tough front surface of your eye. It also preserves the corneal nerve supply, resulting in minimal impact on tear supply during the healing stage. For these reasons it is now offered to all suitable candidates at our practice.

What else is in the pipeline?

Even in these post-GFC times lots of new things are being tried. One company, Nexis Vision (Disclaimer: I'm on their Medical Advisory Board), was started on the premise that if the comfort and speed of recovery in advanced surface laser (ASLA), could be improved to be equivalent to LASIK, then it would dominate. That is definitely true because ASLA is a less expensive option for patients as it requires less disposables and eliminates the need to use a femtosecond laser to cut a flap.

Nexis Vision has produced a soft contact lens which is placed on the surface of the eye, for one week after having ASLA, and during that week of healing they hope that it will provide a level of vision and comfort that allows people to work and drive, similar to what is achieved with LASIK. The pilot trials in the United States have been mixed. It certainly has a long way to go but could potentially be a very interesting development over the next few years and provides an alternative to SMILE laser for lower cost vision correction surgery.

One thing I have learnt over the years is that good ideas come from many, and often unexpected places, so I am always receptive to ideas, but at the same time I look hard at the real data before deciding whether a procedure is sensible to apply to patients.

At the moment, LASIK is still a great option for patients who are anatomically suitable and have the right expectations. SMILE laser appears to offer some advantages over LASIK, especially for certain types of candidate – the dry eye sufferer, the active sportsman – but it is unlikely to be widely available for some time, and to date it caters only for short-sighted eyes. Will SMILE laser supersede LASIK as the new poster child for laser vision correction? Only time will tell.

M.L

DR JOSÉ BARRAQUER

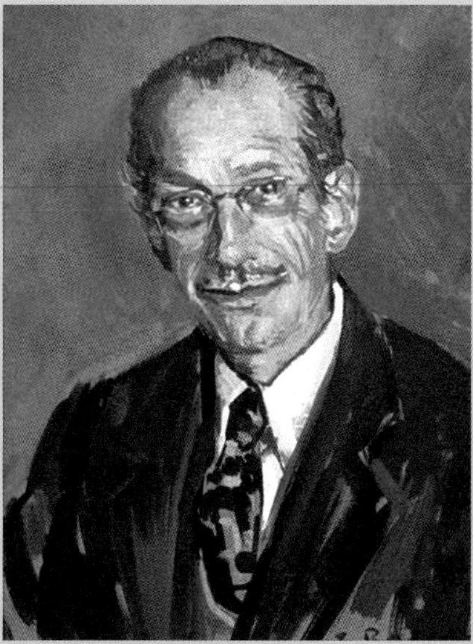

—
José Barraquer

> *One does not discover new lands without consenting to lose sight of the shore for a very long time...*
>
> ***André Gide***

No book on the subject of ophthalmology would be complete without mention of the Barraquer family. Traditionally, the men of the Barraquer family became ophthalmologists and have done this for several generations.

They had (and still have) their own hospital in Barcelona and two of them, José and his brother, Joaquin, both performed their first cataract operation at the age of thirteen. Their father, Ignacio Barraquer, trained them in the art of eye surgery as it was a given that this was what the family did. Whilst Joaquin was very highly regarded as a surgeon, José was considered brilliant.

José Barraquer left the family home in Barcelona and emigrated to Colombia. When he arrived there in 1953 he was thirty-seven years old. Having walked away from his family and the wealth of knowledge and experience they had in ophthalmology, he set about starting all over again. José founded the Barraquer Institute of America and set about revolutionising the world of ophthalmology. He was fascinated with engineering and used this knowledge to develop some startling new operating techniques.

It was in 1947 that José had the original concept that the curvature of the cornea, the clear front of the eye, could be changed optically, like a spectacle or contact lens, to correct the common refractive errors – short-sightedness, long-sightedness and astigmatism. It took him almost 30 years of painstaking research to establish the principles and develop the microsurgical techniques and unique mechanical instrumentation (see below) before he presented his surgical results at the World Corneal Congress II in Washington DC in 1975. Those principles and techniques are still valid for corneal vision correction surgery as it is practiced today with excimer and femtosecond lasers.

José Barraquer invented the procedure known as keratomileusis, which involved shaving off part of the cornea with a mechanised blade he invented, called a microkeratome. He would put the slice of cornea on a special sort of lathe (another invention of his) called a cryolathe, which would freeze it and then mechanically grind it to a new shape before he would put it back on the eye. What he did was mould, or change the shape of the cornea. This was, in effect, the beginning of corneal vision correction surgery. Whilst operating on his own in Bogota, Colombia, in the back blocks of South America, thousands of miles from all the major hospitals, universities and research institutes, José Barraquer developed and refined this unique procedure which brought him international recognition. Keratomileusis was a complex operation and many surgeons travelled to Bogota to learn Barraquer's technique. However, only a small number were able to replicate his results in the USA and Europe and the procedure was reserved for patients with extreme amounts of short-sightedness.

What really mattered were the lessons the profession learnt, e.g. how much the cornea could be altered in shape and still provide good quality vision to the patient.

José Barraquer's success as a surgeon brought him fame and fortune, which in turn brought him to the attention of one of Colombia's left wing guerrilla groups. This was in the late 1970s when one of those periodic waves of killings and kidnappings swept the country. Barraquer was one of a number of high profile Bogota residents who were abducted and ransomed. The negotiations were complex. As a consequence this scion of an incredibly wealthy family in Colombia with links back to Spain remained a hostage while his family and the kidnappers argued about what he was 'worth'. It was five months before the two sides reached agreement and Barraquer was finally released after payment of an undisclosed sum. Luckily for the science of ophthalmology, he was soon back at work.

Understandably, José made some changes to his personal arrangements. When I met and worked with him in Bogota in 1986 I couldn't help but notice that he followed the most extreme security protocols. Each day he travelled to work in one of several different cars – all of which were armour plated. Once in the car park he would remain in the vehicle whilst one of his security-detail walked over and pressed the button for the elevator. When that arrived and opened, only then did Barraquer leave the vehicle and enter the lift. This was 'his' personal elevator – no one else in the building was allowed to use it – it took him from the car park to his clinic and to the laboratory on the top floor. No one was going to kidnap José Barraquer again.

The Barraquer Institute of America included its own hospital, which is where I spent two months learning all that I could. A group of about a dozen of us did the rounds of the hospital with him. One day we came to the bedside of a patient who had undergone a cataract procedure the day before. Barraquer was not at all physically imposing. He was a grey old man, very quiet – didn't say much. To me he seemed to have this unusual combination of possessing the brain of a great engineer and a great clinician. Many of the instruments we developed he built himself.

In those days the surgeon would sometimes leave a small amount of air inside the eye in order to protect the structures. Barraquer examined his patient and then turned to our group and pointed at me. "You! Michael!" he exclaimed in English. "There is too much air in this eye. What would you do?" Quickly I thought about it and replied, "Well, I would take the patient to the slit lamp (the microscope) and measure the pressure. If I felt there was too much air, I'd insert a very fine needle through the edge and extract this small amount of air. You wouldn't have to take it all out, just a small amount."

As I explained myself and not all that confidently, Barraquer stood there listening and nodding. After I finished there was a silence. I wondered if I had said the wrong thing, or if I should say more. Not knowing what to do, I added as confidently as I could, "That's how I would do it."

Barraquer looked at me. "Huh," was all he said. Then he leaned over the patient lying in the bed, and pressed on the eye with his thumb. Out popped the trapped air. "This is how I would do it!" Barraquer announced with a flourish.

In 1982 Barraquer teamed up with Dr Richard (Dick) Troutman, a New York-based world expert of corneal transplantation and close associate. Together they formed the International Society of Refractive Surgery which was soon at the forefront of education in the burgeoning field of vision correction. José Barraquer was the first President of that Society. He died in 1998 at the age of eighty-two. Today, he is considered by many to have been "the father" of modern vision correction surgery.
The Barraquer Institute still exists in Bogota. It is now run by his daughter, Carmen Barraquer. ●

G.S

THE BEAUTY OF BLENDED VISION

The real voyage of discovery consists not in seeking new landscapes, but in having new eyes.
Marcel Proust, Remembrance of Things Past

If you're over fifty, you are not going to get a vision correction surgery result that gives you back the vision you had when you were thirty. It's as simple as that. Your eyes change in your mid-forties and need some extra help with focusing up close. So, we get around that problem for our patients by providing a new way of seeing. It's called **blended vision** and that's how my eyes work since I've had my own procedure. My dominant (right) eye sees clearly in the distance and my perception is that my distance vision is clear with both eyes. It feels normal. However, if I cover my right eye and look in the distance it is a bit blurred. I have deliberately left my left eye a bit short-sighted so that it can help me out with most of my reading tasks. Certainly using a computer, reading patient files, and all the general day-to-day stuff is fine for me without glasses. But there is some compromise. I have a pair of glasses that I use for reading in poor light.

It is a fact that some people expect too much from blended vision. They want the sun, the moon and the stars.

This blended vision option is very successful for most people. At the initial consultation, we give our patients a 'test-drive', where they try out the end result by wearing a pair of ultra-thin, comfortable soft contact lenses for an hour or two. Our staff put the lenses in and you would barely notice they were there, they are so comfortable. It allows you to go for a coffee or a walk and trial what your vision would be like if you had the blended vision procedure. Most people love it and they accept the compromise. But, like everything else in life, it's not for everyone. We even give our over-forty-five-year-old patients a questionnaire where they have to rate their own personality type on a scale that goes from 'easy-going' on one end to 'perfectionist' on the other!

It is a fact that some people expect too much from blended vision. They want the sun, the moon and the stars. They want excellent vision at all distances and they are not willing to accept any compromise. It's just part of their psyche. Hollywood film director Bruce Beresford is a classic example of this.

CASE STUDY

I can tell you about Bruce as a patient because he has published a terrific memoir, *Josh Hartnett Definitely Wants To Do This ... True Stories From A Life In The Screen Trade*, in which he details his experience as my patient.

Bruce is an interesting character. He came to see me about laser surgery some years ago and I realised very quickly that I was dealing with a perfectionist.

Bruce is an interesting character. He came to see me about laser surgery some years ago and I realised very quickly that I was dealing with a perfectionist. He was well over fifty at the time, and what he wanted was what everyone wants – to be able to improve his distance vision, but also sufficiently improve his near vision so that he could read a script without glasses. He wanted to be able to go to a movie set or use a computer and not have to wear glasses. The only way to achieve that is with a blended vision correction so that one eye is a bit better for distance and one eye is a bit better for near. We started as we always do by trialling that effect with contact lenses of various different strengths and after much experimentation, Bruce eventually decided on the blended vision 'mix' he wanted.

I did the surgery and obtained a perfect result of exactly what we had targeted. He went back to his optometrist, and the optometrist sent me a letter back saying that Bruce was exactly on target but had changed his mind in terms of what he wanted. The reading vision was terrific but he wanted a little bit less reading vision and wanted to be able to see in the middle distance so he could see the expressions on the actors' faces. He said that that was just not quite good enough. As a film director he needed to see the nuance.

Bruce was quite unlike any other patient of mine. While he was overseas, he sent me a postcard about once a week. "Dear Gerard," he would report, "My eyes are still not quite right."

I said, "Okay, we can make an adjustment, but I want you to be sure of it." Bruce explained that he was leaving to shoot a film in Eastern Europe. We agreed to just leave it for the moment and he could use a pair of glasses. He would let me know how things were going, and on his return I would do an enhancement procedure.

I have to say, Bruce was quite unlike any other patient of mine. While he was overseas, he sent me a postcard about once a week. "Dear Gerard," he would report, "My eyes are still not quite right." Bruce would then detail his experience on set and where he was having problems.

When he returned to Australia he had an enhancement and has been very happy ever since. In fact, Bruce has sent me a lot of people from the film industry. I saw his daughter and did surgery on her.

Then, out of the blue one day he sent me a note – "Dear Gerard, just to let you know, I have written a book and you are in it." He might have even sent me a copy. I was really excited, if a bit nervous. I opened the book and searched high and low and eventually found in the entry for October…, "I saw Dr Sutton again. He finally gets my eyes right." That was to me just a classic example of Bruce's sense of humour. Sometimes, even with the nicest people, you can get a situation where you get a result that is spot on but due to a shift in expectations you need to get them back and tweak it a bit. We now call this at our practice, the 'Beresford Effect' … I have a feeling that Bruce would approve. ●

—
Bruce Beresford (centre), John Cusack and Morgan Freeman on set of The Contract *(2006) reproduced with kind permission from Bruce Beresford*

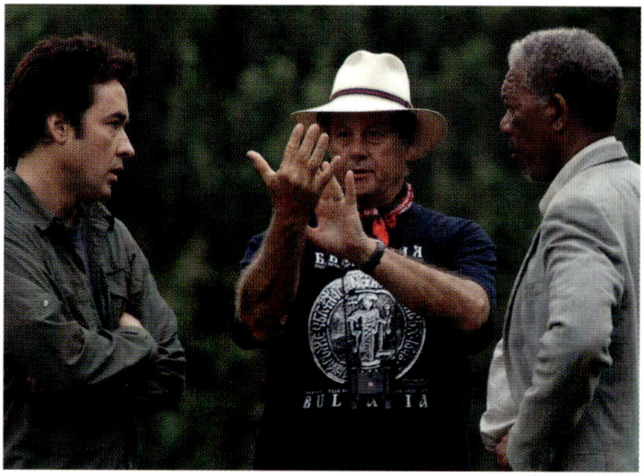

M.L

DR SVYATOSLAV FYODOROV

Every now and then a man's mind is stretched by a new idea or sensation, and never shrinks back to its former dimensions.

Oliver Wendell Holmes,
American physician, poet and essayist

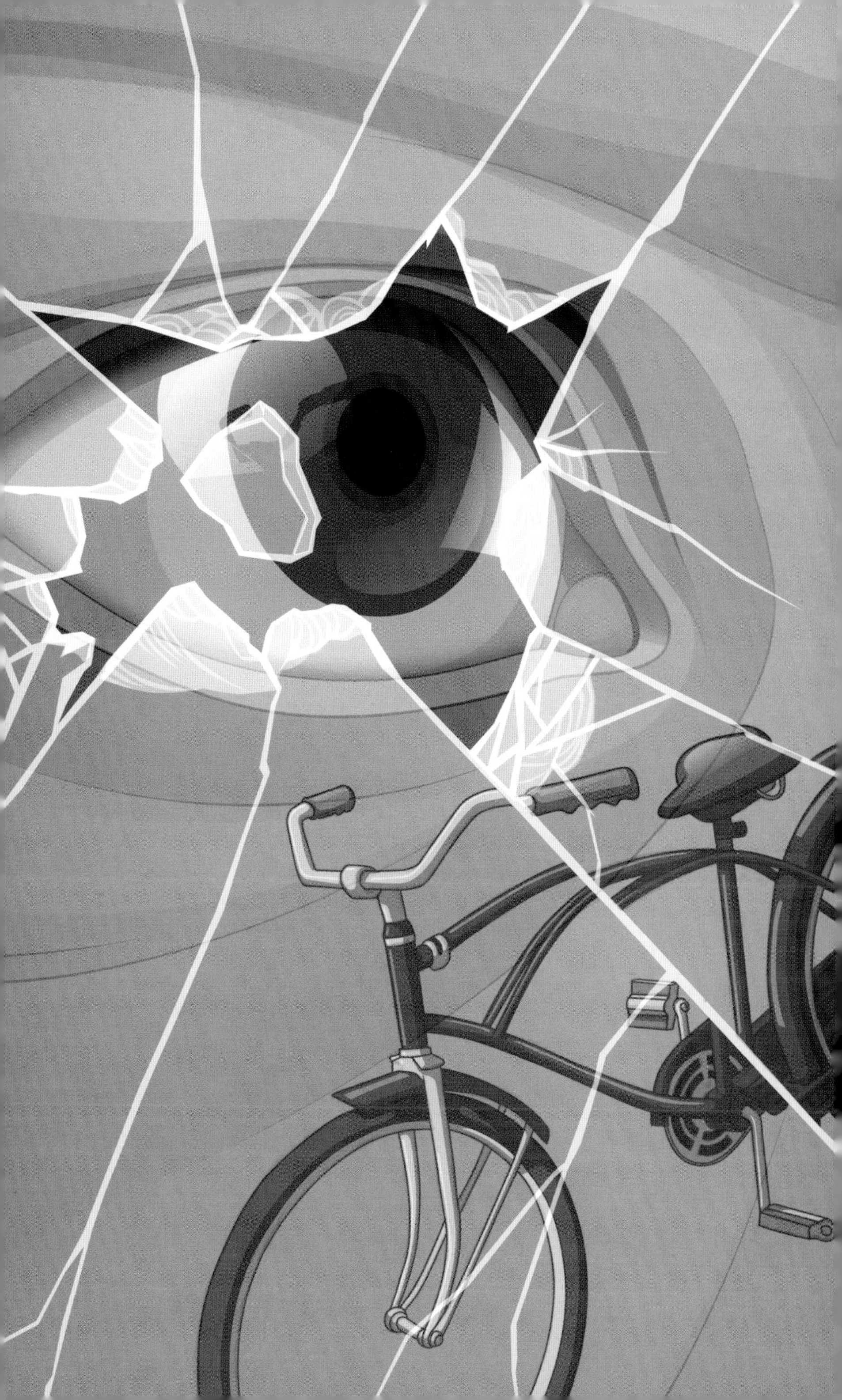

The history of ophthalmology has often been driven by some very eccentric geniuses, none more so than Svyatoslav Nikolayevich Fyodorov. An astonishing individual by any measure, Fyodorov was responsible for some of the greatest advances ever made in the field of corrective surgery. Born in the Ukraine in 1927, Fyodorov worked as an ophthalmologist in a small town in Rostov Oblast. In 1973 he developed a new surgical technique, called scleroplasty, to cure the early stages of glaucoma.

One day in 1974, a fifteen-year-old boy presented as a patient. His problem was unusual. He'd fallen from his bicycle and some pieces of glass had gone into one eye. For whatever reason, the boy received no medical treatment and although he appeared to have recovered, he now complained that one eye was different to the other. It was presumed that the glass had damaged the cornea of one eye and, as it had been untreated, now affected his vision.

When Fyodorov examined the boy's eyes, what he saw was to lead to the greatest revolution in eye surgery in hundreds of years. One eye, the boy's uninjured eye, was still short-sighted -3.00 or -4.00. The other eye, which had been cut by the piece of glass externally, had healed with a scar, yet incredibly the optical error had been fixed. He was no longer short-sighted in this eye. Fyodorov realised that the glass had cut the cornea, then healed in a way that flattened the cornea and fixed the short-sightedness in that eye. Obviously Fyodorov knew of Sato's work in Japan and with this discovery he now realised that Sato was almost right – he just did his procedure from the wrong direction. Thanks to doctors like Sato we now understand that the back of the cornea really matters. Fyodorov realised that corrective surgery on the cornea would work if the surgeon came in from the front.

What this bit of glass had done to this Russian boy's eye was what Fyodorov now began to experiment with, and in the process invented a procedure now known as radial keratotomy (RK) – 'radial' meaning radiating out (like the spokes of a bicycle wheel) and 'keratotomy' meaning cuts to the cornea (the front surface of the eye).

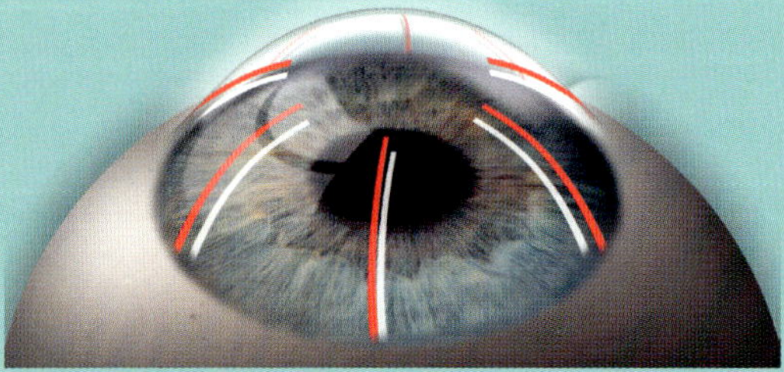

The red lines show the position of the cuts Fyodorov made to the front surface of the cornea in the procedure known as ***Radial Keratotomy****. The white lines show the position of the cuts made decades earlier by Japanese Dr Sato to the back surface of the cornea.*

In a way Fyodorov was the catalyst for my decision to become an ophthalmologist. I was an intern at Royal Newcastle Hospital and while doing some notes in the on-call room I overheard a story on the radio about this brilliant Russian doctor who had invented this new operation which in all likelihood would solve the problem of short-sightedness for millions of people. As I listened to this news report I was transfixed and thought this was the most phenomenal achievement. Never in my wildest dreams did I imagine that I would actually meet Fyodorov and many of the world's leading ophthalmologists and surgeons.

Also, it has to be remembered that Fyodorov's break-through occurred at the height of the Cold War and for doctors in the West it was almost inconceivable that an unknown provincial specialist in a 'renegade' state like the Soviet Union could do this. However, it soon became apparent that Fyodorov was the real deal and although a group of American ophthalmologists brought scientific rigour to radial keratotomy he was universally recognised as the creator of this procedure. It was the American doctors who worked out the size of incisions, how deep they should be, whether you should use a diamond blade, rather than a metal blade, how to modify the healing, and so on. A great deal was learnt as hundreds of thousands of radial keratotomy procedures were done, mostly with quite good results.

By any measure, Fyodorov was an exceptional human being. As he was intrigued by time and motion studies, he developed a form of automated surgery. Fyodorov developed hospitals where the surgeon would sit in one place and the patient would be placed on a conveyor belt bed which would move in front of the surgeon. The doctor would perform his operation and at the conclusion of the procedure the bed would rotate out and be replaced by the next patient. He also organised a series of 'hospital' ships – the idea being that patients from western countries could have their eye operations while sailing the Mediterranean. It was never a great success. Fyodorov was a far better doctor than he was a businessman.

In the 1980s Fyodorov was appointed head of the Moscow Research Institute of Eye Microsurgery and when the communist government collapsed he was elected a member of the Russian parliament. I met him a number of times at medical conferences in the United States. Physically, Fyodorov was an imposing presence even though he lost a foot in an accident shortly after finishing high school.

Fyodorov ran for the Presidency of Russia in the 1991 and 1996 elections, standing against Boris Yeltsin, but was not successful. Sadly, he was killed in a helicopter crash in the year 2000. In 2001, when I was President of the Society of Refractive Surgery, I hosted a table with his children and his family at a dinner. The Fyodorov family believed that there were grave doubts as to whether the helicopter crash was a genuine accident. They suspected that he had been murdered by his enemies. Fyodorov's death was a tragedy for modern medicine, but his legacy lives on. ●

M.L

LASER LENS SURGERY

Laser lens surgery is increasingly becoming the vision correction procedure of choice for our over-55 year old patients. As its safety profiles and the predictability of its outcomes approach those of LASIK, ASLA and SMILE laser, lens replacement surgery has enjoyed a surge in popularity.

Lens replacement surgery offers a number of advantages over LASIK, ASLA and SMILE laser for the carefully chosen patient. Not only do you have your lenses replaced for once and for all, eliminating the need to ever undergo cataract surgery, you also have a wider range of options to correct presbyopia – the deterioration of reading vision that comes on with increasing age. The advent of multifocal and trifocal intraocular lenses now allows a more natural way of seeing, post-surgery, than older intraocular designs provided.

In all lens replacement surgery, the eye's natural lens is gently removed and replaced with an artificial lens, which has been carefully selected for your individual needs to minimise dependence on glasses. While a LASIK, ASLA or SMILE laser procedure on your cornea cannot give us a multifocal or trifocal option, this can be achieved with an artificial lens, if desired. Alternatively, a blended vision outcome can be created.

Until very recently, most aspects of lens replacement surgery – including the initial incision, the opening of the lens capsule and the break-up of the eye's natural lens – were performed manually by the surgeon. Technology is constantly improving and with the introduction of the latest laser lens surgery technique, several of these manual steps can now be performed with the high-precision femtosecond laser. I was very fortunate to be in the position to perform the first laser lens procedure in the country in April 2011 using the femtosecond laser, and both Gerard and I are firm advocates of its advantages over older techniques and now perform all lens replacement surgery in this way.

Femtosecond Technology

Until very recently, most aspects of lens replacement surgery, including the initial incision, the opening of the lens capsule and the break-up of the eye's crystalline lens, were performed manually by the surgeon. Technology is constantly improving and with the introduction of the latest Laser Lens Surgery technique, several of these manual steps can now be performed with the high-precision femtosecond laser. The creation of the incision, the separation of the circle of tissue on the lens surface and then the breakup of the core material inside the lens were all manual steps that are now done with the femtosecond laser. I was very fortunate at our practice to be in the position to perform the very first **Laser Lens Surgery** procedure in the country in April 2011 using the **femtosecond laser**, and both Gerard and I are firm advocates of its advantages over older techniques and now perform lens replacement surgery in this way for the majority of our patients.

The lens replacement procedure – step by step

Step 1. We dilate your iris to get it out of the way, like pushing back a pair of curtains. We use a simple eye drop to do this. Then we can see the underlying lens, your own natural lens, a little jelly-like disc that sits behind your iris.

Step 2. Next, to get access to the inside of the eye, we need to make a tiny incision – only 2.2mm wide – near the edge of your cornea. It acts like a tiny port through which the surgical instruments can enter the eye. It is

The manual creation of the corneal incision with a diamond blade.

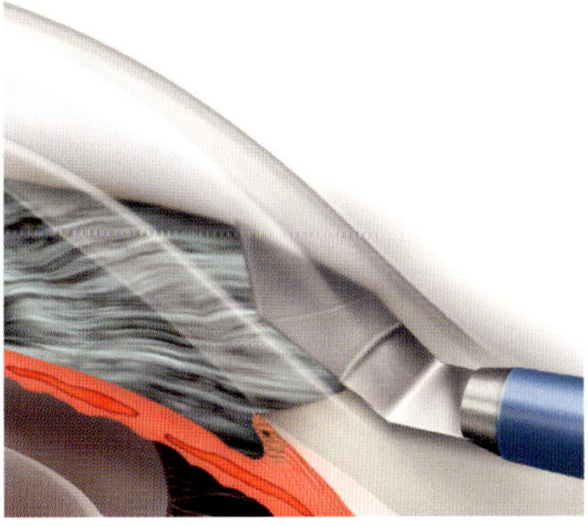

The corneal incision is specially shaped to self-seal.

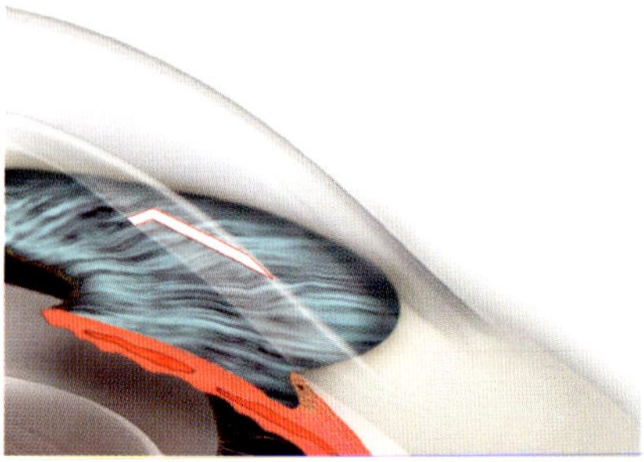

Traditionally, access to the contents of the lens was gained by manually tearing a circle of tissue with a tiny forceps.

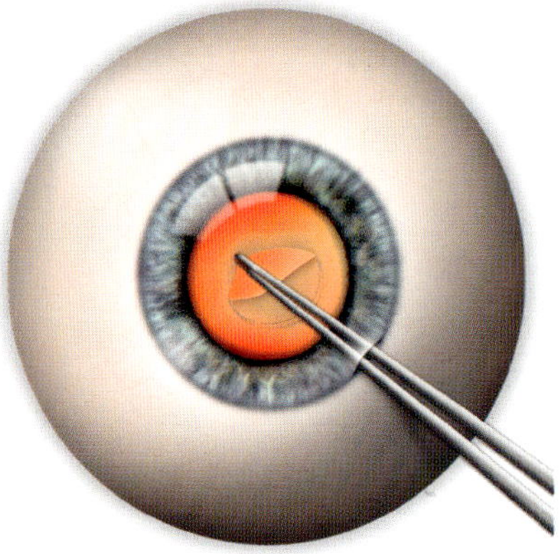

called a clear incision and the nice thing about it is that there is no bleeding because there are no blood vessels in your cornea.

This incision, traditionally performed with a diamond blade, is a special type of incision. It's like a trapdoor, so when we slide the diamond blade through the cornea it doesn't go straight in; it goes in at a steep angle and it changes direction. The beauty of this kind of incision is that when the procedure is over and the instruments are removed, the incision just seals itself shut due to the forces of pressure inside the eye. It doesn't even need a single suture (or stitch). The incision just closes like a perfect seal and doesn't allow any nasties (bacteria etc.) in or any fluid out – one of the many little miracles of modern microsurgery.

With a femtosecond laser there is no need for an incision to be made using a diamond blade. Instead, tiny pulses of energy from the laser create a series of overlapping spaces in the cornea and this gives us access to the eye without having to use a blade to make an incision. As well as improved precision, it allows the incision shape to provide something that a blade cannot; the most favoured incision is now what is called reverse trapezoidal, slightly larger internally than externally. This allows for less stress on the wound during the procedure and, in theory, leads to a more secure wound post-operatively.

Step 3. The next step in the lens replacement procedure involves getting access to the material inside your lens. Your natural lens consists of three layers; a skin (or capsule) a core (or nucleus) and the main body of the lens (the cortex). The capsule needs to have a circle of tissue removed from its front surface to allow access to the cortex within. This procedure is called a capsulotomy. It was traditionally done by hand so we would literally, with a tiny pair of forceps, grab hold of the tissue, pinch it and tear it around in a perfect little circle and then pull it out through this tiny incision. It is an incredibly skilful procedure that takes us years to perfect.

The femtosecond laser creates the circular access to the underlying lens material without an instrument ever touching the eye.

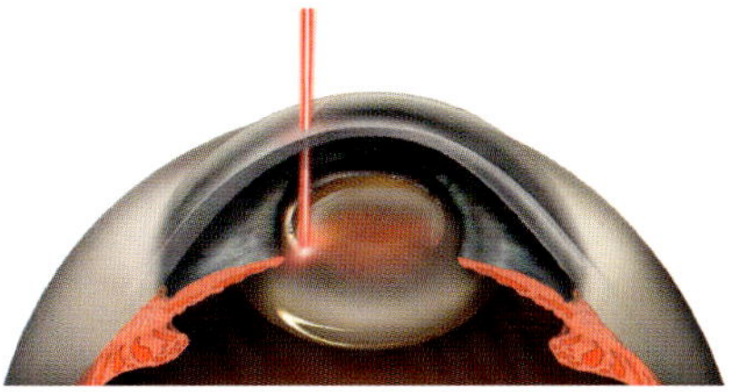

This is the single most critical step in cataract surgery. If the section of tissue removed is round, of the correct diameter and perfectly positioned, it leads to safer surgery by minimising the risk of tears to the capsule, and also allows for the artificial lens to be placed in a more stable position. This has already been shown in previous studies to produce clinical benefits.

The surgeon removes the circle of capsular tissue that has been created by the femtosecond laser.

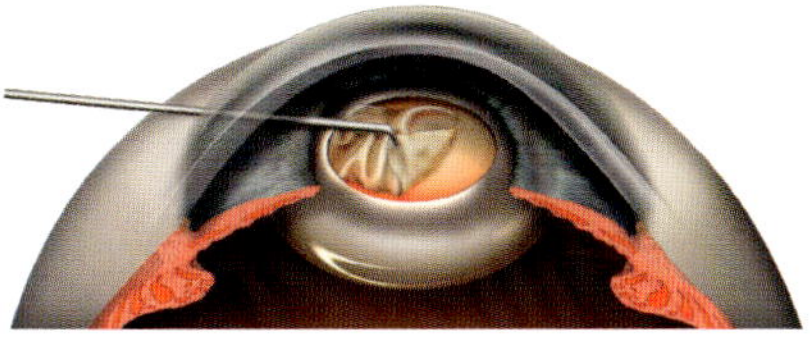

This step can now also performed using the femtosecond laser. The laser separates the circle of capsular tissue from the lens so that the surgeon just has to pull it away and remove it from the eye.

The lens material is broken up and vacuumed out of the eye, leaving the capsule intact.

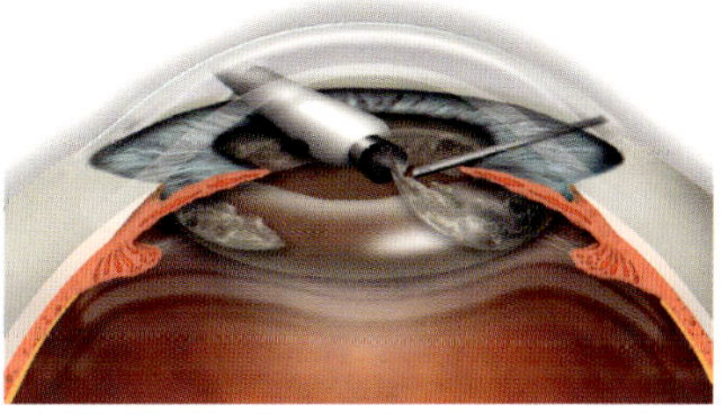

Step 4. The next step involves the removal of the contents of the lens. (It can be useful to think of your lens as a bit like a candy-coated chocolate such as a Smartie or M&M… The candy-coated shell is like our lens capsule, while the chocolate inside is like the cortex and nucleus of our lens. We want to remove all of the chocolate whilst leaving the candy shell perfectly intact apart from a circular access hatch at the front). The contents of the crystalline lens

are removed through a special tool which works a bit like a tiny vacuum cleaner. It provides energy and also vacuums out the lens material through the tiny incision. But the lens capsule (or skin) is left intact. It is attached quite firmly with little tiny fibres – called zonules – to the rest of the eye. These are tiny spoke-like threads right around the lens connecting it to the eye, and if you take the whole lens out (as was standard practice many years ago) you can risk retinal detachment or a retinal tear. It disrupts the whole eye. So by leaving the capsule intact, not only does it avoid disrupting the rest of the eye but it also provides the perfect place to pop your intraocular lens inside.

The tightly folded artificial lens is injected into the empty lens capsule

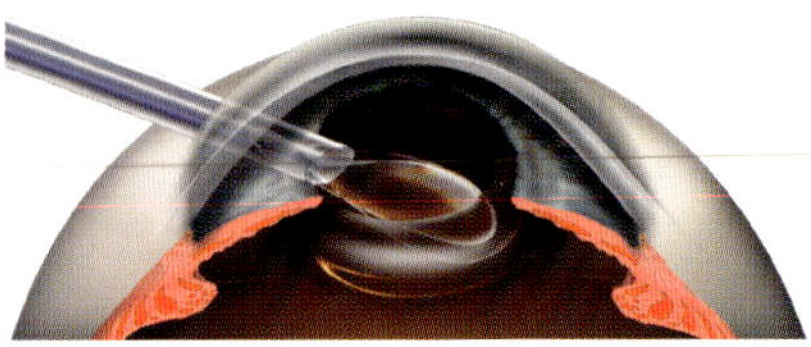

The artificial lens unfolds into place with its struts holding it in position

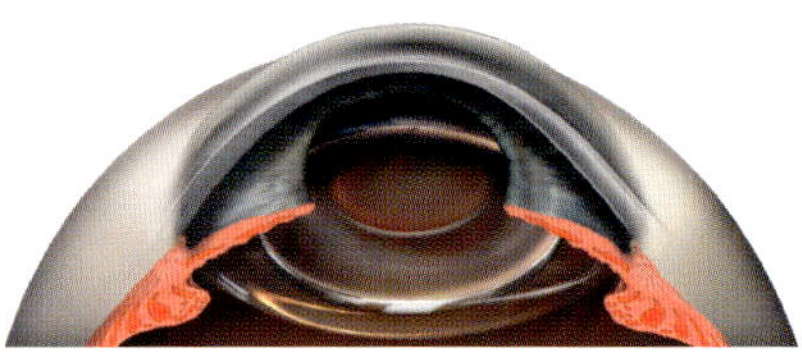

The third thing that the femtosecond laser does is it actually starts to fragment and soften the material inside the lens ready for extraction. Dividing the centre of the lens with the laser means that the time taken for this part of the procedure can be reduced by about 50%. This means less risk of damage to the lens capsule and to the back surface of the cornea.

Step 5. Then we place an artificial lens inside the empty capsule. This artificial lens is specifically chosen for you from a huge bank of lenses so that it will give you the best possible outcome in terms of freedom from glasses. Current artificial lenses are much smaller than our natural lens and they are held in place by tiny struts which sit in the recesses of the now empty lens capsule and hold the artificial lens in a central position. (Once your iris constricts back to normal after the surgery and makes a nice small pupil again, you can't see the intra-ocular lens anymore because it is hidden behind your iris). During this stage of the surgery, a tiny syringe is inserted which squeezes the tightly rolled-up artificial lens into the empty capsule. The artificial lens emerges from the syringe and opens up – you can imagine it a bit like a butterfly emerging from a chrysalis

– and its little placement struts (acting like springs) sit into the inside of the capsule to hold it in position.

In conclusion

It is tempting to think of lens replacement surgery as a simple procedure; no stitches, no injections, just a single drop of local anaesthetic to numb the eye… But it is certainly not simple. It is a highly complex procedure, but due to the beautiful microsurgery technique it causes very little trauma to the eye and yet achieves such a profound effect. You can think about it like this: the easier it is for the eye, the trickier it is for the surgeon.

Lens replacement surgery is used all over the world to replace lenses that have become clouded with cataract. As vision correction surgeons we use it more and more to correct vision in people who don't have cataracts but are simply seeking freedom from glasses. **Laser Lens Surgery** (using the femtosecond laser) is increasingly becoming the vision correction procedure of choice for our over-55 year old patients. As safety profiles and predictability of outcomes approach those of LASIK, ASLA and SMILE, lens replacement surgery has enjoyed a surge in popularity. It offers a number of advantages over these corneal procedures for the carefully-chosen patient. Not only do you have your lenses replaced for once and for all, eliminating the need to ever undergo cataract surgery, you also have a wider range of options to correct presbyopia – the deterioration of reading vision that comes on with increasing age. The advent of multifocal / trifocal intraocular lenses now allows a more natural way of seeing, post-surgery, than older intraocular designs provided.

As safety profiles and predictability of outcomes approach those of LASIK, ASLA and SMILE, lens replacement surgery has enjoyed a surge in popularity. It offers a number of advantages over these corneal procedures for the carefully-chosen patient.

There is significant extra cost (to surgeon and patient) in having lens replacement performed with the femtosecond laser rather than manually, but we believe that the benefits are clear. Laser Lens Surgery performs those three important steps with a precision and reproducibility that is not possible with the human hand, no matter how steady or experienced. Laser Lens Surgery has been available in Australia since April 2011 and we now perform the vast majority of lens replacement surgery in this way. There is emerging evidence that it is a safer way to perform the procedure and achieves a better result.

CASE STUDY

Jenny is fifty-eight when she first comes to see me, although I have to say, she looks a lot younger. She wears glasses for distance and near vision and also wears contact lenses when she can manage them. As she is long-sighted (about +3 for distance, + 5.50 for reading), she explains that it is difficult for her to actually see the contact lenses on her finger-tip, in order to put them into her eyes correctly. They are always popping inside-out or falling to the floor, so they are reserved for social occasions – of which it sounds like there are many. Most of the time she wears glasses and shows me that her bag is chock full of glasses, several pairs of which seem to be designer sunglasses. Jenny's eyes are healthy on examination with nothing out of the ordinary. She does have a mild dry-eye condition, which is very common in post-menopausal women, but as she is able to wear her soft lenses comfortably, I don't see her dry eye as a show-stopper. If she proceeded with a LASIK procedure we would ensure that she had plenty of support from artificial tears during the healing period.

It is difficult for her to actually see the contact lenses on her finger-tip, in order to put them into her eyes correctly. They are always popping inside-out or falling to the floor, so they are reserved for social occasions

We discuss all the vision correction options and although LASIK is an option for her, she is very interested in the idea of laser lens surgery with multifocal lenses. This is a more invasive procedure than LASIK but also extremely successful and safe, with very

So, what can you expect if you have a laser vision correction procedure on your lens?

This is what we advise our patients:

- On the day of your lens procedure you will spend about 2 to 3 hours in our specialised day surgery.
- Modern lens surgery is performed under local anaesthesia to numb your eye so there is no need for a general anaesthetic or an over-night hospital stay. You will be made very comfortable for your procedure with a gentle intravenous sedative and there is rarely any discomfort or pain during the procedure.
- After your procedure you will be provided with refreshments and your eye may be gently covered with an eye-shield to allow safe healing overnight.
- You return to our centre the next day to have the vision assessed.
- You will be given special medicated eye drops to use according to your surgeon's instructions for a few weeks after your procedure. These antibiotic and anti-inflammatory eye drops protect the eye during the important healing process.
- You will be advised to avoid strenuous activities and water in your eyes for the first few days after surgery. Most normal daily activities can be resumed within a day or two and your surgeon will instruct you on when you may resume contact sports etc.
- You should always advise your surgeon or the clinic promptly if there is pain, redness of the eye or blurring of vision during the early days or weeks after surgery.
- Your eyes will be examined several times during the first few weeks after surgery. You may experience excellent vision as early as the next day after your procedure or it may take a little longer (typically days to weeks) to settle, during which time your vision may fluctuate.
- All eye surgery has the potential for complications that may affect your vision. However, lens surgery is one of the safest operations that can be undertaken and most complications, while rare, can be remedied with further treatment.

low risk of complications in a healthy eye. LASIK could offer Jenny a blended vision result where one eye would be clearer for distance and the other eye clearer for near vision (see page 82 for more information on blended vision). However, as LASIK is a corneal procedure, it would mean that down the track, Jenny could require further eye surgery should cataracts develop in her natural lenses with increasing age. One of the advantages of a lens procedure for Jenny would be that her natural lenses would be replaced once and once only, so she would never have to worry about the trouble or expense of cataract surgery in the future. Once your lenses are replaced you will never develop a cataract. The other advantage of having a lens procedure instead of a corneal procedure like LASIK is the option of multifocal intraocular lenses. When your natural lenses are removed, we replace them with tiny artificial lenses called intraocular lenses and these come in many wonderful designs, including multifocal options which provide clear vision for both distance and near for both eyes.

Scientists are trying to make a polymer that is identical to our lens and can flex like our lens and behave like our lens – before it loses its flexibility.

Multifocal intraocular lenses are not for everyone. Depending on how strong you want the reading vision to be, they may involve some compromise to the quality and 'crispness' of your distance vision, most obviously for tasks such as night driving. But they do have some marvellous benefits, such as the ability to see with both eyes at a range of distances. This type of procedure is ideal for someone with vision that is already slightly compromised, due to the development of early-stage cataracts, for example, or even someone who doesn't wear their glasses as much as they should and is used to a slight compromise in their vision. Also, personality comes into play in determining if multifocal lens surgery is the best choice of procedure. It is best suited to people with an easy-going disposition. We try and avoid recommending them to those who already have exceptional vision with their glasses and might be perfectionists! The thing is, if you are a very fussy type and you are used to crystal clear vision through your glasses, it is difficult to adjust to any sort of compromise, even if you have the huge upside of independence from glasses brought about by vision correction surgery.

From a long discussion with Jenny, I was confident that she would love the results of multifocal lens surgery. We scheduled her procedures one week apart and even from the first post-operative visit she was very positive about the outcome, even though it took her a few months to fully adjust to her distance vision for night driving. She confided in me that she uses it as an excuse to not be the designated driver ... That's an advantage for having multifocal intraocular lenses which had never occurred to me.

And the future? The artificial lenses used in lens replacement surgery are made of synthetic materials called polymers. These polymers are heavier than our natural lens. We haven't to date been able to exactly mimic the material that our own natural lenses are made from. That's where a lot of the research is now focused. Scientists are trying to make a polymer that is identical to our lens and can flex like our lens and behave like our lens – before it loses its flexibility. What happens is that as we age our lens become harder and less flexible – this is especially noticeable when you get into your mid-forties. That is the future of lens replacement surgery – where we use a polymer that behaves exactly like your own natural lens so we could remove your lens and put in this polymer instead. Will they achieve this nirvana in my life-time? You never know! ●

G.S THE INVENTION OF LASER EYE SURGERY

While a handful of pioneers started a revolution in vision correction surgery, their techniques relied on mechanically altering the cornea using blades and lathes. This was all to change with the discovery of an unusual application of the excimer laser.

An American ophthalmologist, Steve Trokel, enjoyed the unique hobby of spending his down time leafing through volume upon volume of unclassified US Military data on military experiments. He was well aware that the US Military devotes massive resources in the pursuit of new technology to give its forces superior weaponry systems. Occasionally, these inventions have a civilian spin-off. The classic example being the GPS system which was designed by the US Department of Defence as a navigation tool for guided missiles and today just about everyone has one in their car.

One day in 1982 Steve Trokel came across a report where scientists had been using excimer lasers on the corneas of laboratory rabbits – just why they were conducting such research was a mystery never explained. Excimer lasers were originally used in the 1970s by IBM for etching silicone computer chips. What excited Trokel was that when he examined photographs of the experiments he noticed that the lasers had shaved the corneas of the rabbits without damaging the surrounding tissue. When the military scientists used an excimer laser at the particular wavelength of 193 nanometres, they could remove corneal tissue with extreme precision and more remarkably, with no collateral damage to the cornea. Trokel thought this was unbelievable. He understood lasers and thought it was inconceivable that they would not harm the eye. When a surgeon uses a scalpel in radial keratotomy it cuts the cornea, which later heals with a scar. The laser was changing the cornea's shape, but otherwise not affecting it at all.

Trokel knew that the only way to understand what was happening was to conduct his own experiments. He and his colleagues gained access to an excimer laser, set it at exactly 193 nanometres and zapped the corneas of laboratory rabbits. In 1983 Trokel's paper, describing how it was possible to use a laser to permanently change the shape of the cornea without damaging it, was published in the American Journal of Ophthalmology. And so it was that this random result of a military experiment on rabbits became the catalyst for modern-day laser vision correction.

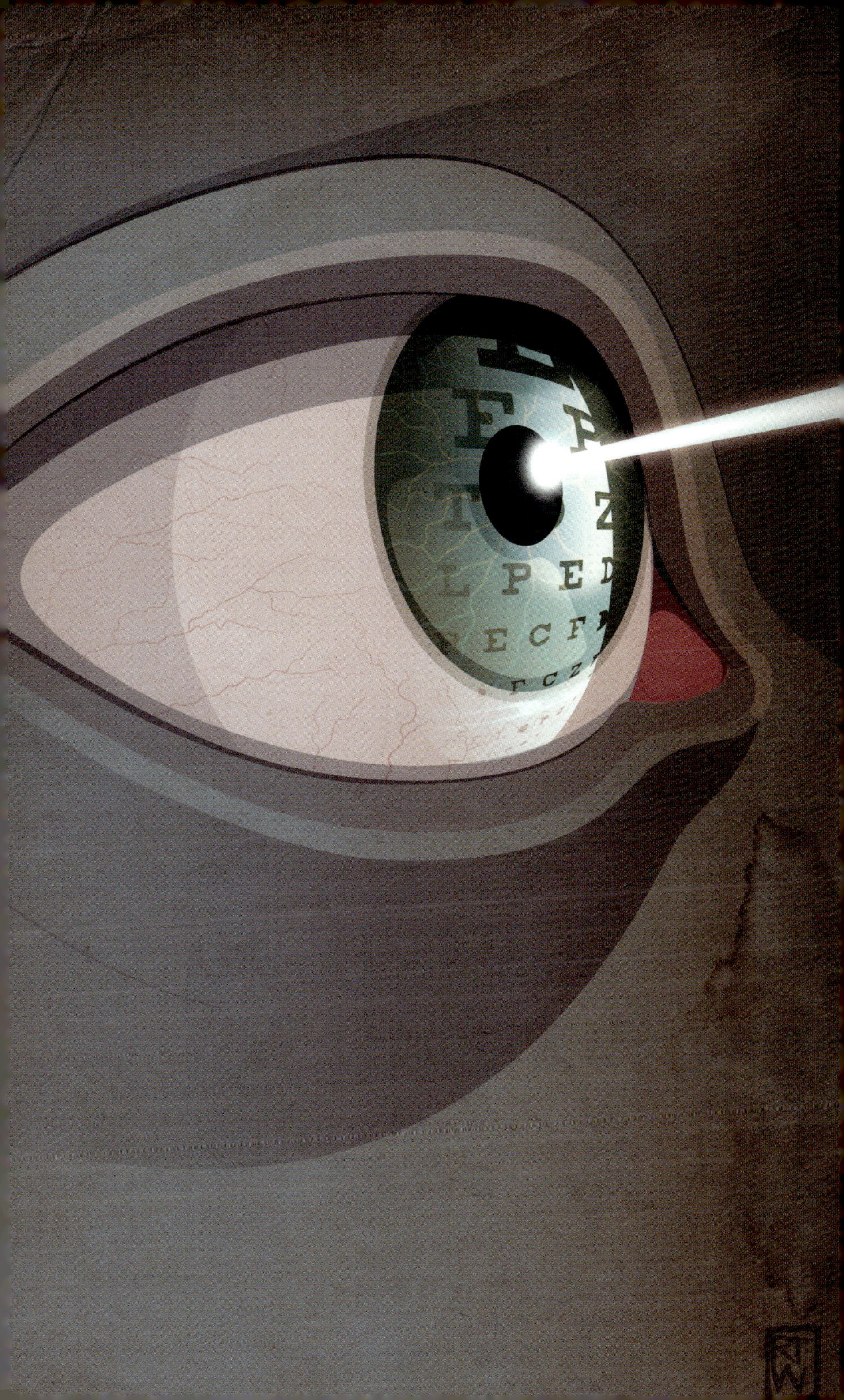
L P E D

In Germany, Dr Theo Seiler recognised the significance of Trokel's discovery. Within two years Seiler had reached the stage with his independent research where he was confident enough to use the excimer laser to cut the cornea of a human cadaver eye. Thus the first procedure on a human eye with the excimer laser happened in Dresden, Germany in 1985.

Seiler showed that it could be done, but the hard work was not over yet. Trokel and his colleagues in the US worked closely with Professor John Marshall of London for many years. During the early to mid-1980s Trokel took an overnight plane every month from the US to London to see Marshall, who would study the specimens he brought with him. These specimens were of two types – those with radial excisions (like RK) and those with a central disc of tissue removed. At the time it was controversial to remove corneal tissue from the central part of the cornea because of the risk of scarring but these studies established that the corneas did not scar.

By the mid-1980s, Marshall recognised that the corneal tissue needed to be removed in a smooth disc shape (known as a lenticular cut), which would sculpt the whole cornea, rather than the discrete radial cuts that Trokel and Seiler had initially been focusing on. They had essentially been replicating the Radial Keratotomy techniques with a laser instead of a blade. This was a huge leap forward and Marshall was awarded a patent on the technique, which was known as Photo Refractive Keratectomy (better known as PRK, and today as ASLA).

In 1988, in New Orleans, USA, Dr Marguerite McDonald performed the first PRK procedure in the world on a patient's healthy eye. This was essentially the beginning of laser eye surgery. Some forty years after Dr Barraquer's first trials of his vision correction procedure, Trokel, Marshall, McDonald and their colleagues used the excimer laser directly on the outermost layers of the cornea to treat short-sightedness.

Michael Lawless followed those scientific breakthroughs with great interest and planned with Dr Chris Rogers (and later Dr Peter Cohen) to bring an excimer laser to Australia. In September 1991 Dr Peter Cohen did the first PRK procedure in the country and Chris and Michael did their first operations a couple of days later. That same year Dr Geoffrey Crawford and Dr Graham Barrett in Perth also started treating patients with an excimer laser that had been developed in conjunction with the Lions Eye Institute.

Although PRK was effective at treating low to moderate levels of short-sightedness and led to good outcomes, it wasn't as successful with higher prescriptions, where it led to a greater incidence of corneal haze and loss of corrected visual acuity. On top of that, it was pretty uncomfortable for the patient during the healing period and that, along with the delay in visual recovery (sometimes several weeks) meant that widespread acceptance of PRK remained elusive.

In 1990 Dr Ioannis Pallikaris of Crete decided that PRK was too painful for the patient, that the recovery period was too slow, and that healing was a bit too unpredictable for his liking. Pallikaris experimented with the idea of doing the laser procedure under a little flap or layer of the cornea. He cut a layer with a bladed instrument (called a microkeratome), lifted up the flap, used the laser to reshape the underlying corneal tissue and then put the layer back. No sutures or stitches – the cornea sealed itself. Thus, Pallikaris invented and named the procedure we now know as LASIK – Laser in-situ keratomileusis. The procedure was gradually refined so that by 1995 its use became widespread. It was everything he had hoped for: it was more comfortable for the patient, their recovery was quicker, and the healing more controlled. Pallikaris wasn't the only one who recognised that Barraquer's technique of sculpting the cornea *away* from the surface of the eye was the way forward, especially as they could now do it with a laser instead of a cryolathe. Dr Lucio Burrato in Milan independently invented a technique of creating a disc of corneal tissue with a microkeratome and, in a technique very similar to Barraquer's cryolathing, he used the excimer laser to reshape the back surface of the disc before suturing it back into place on the cornea. However, it wasn't as effective as Pallikaris' technique, which has endured to this day, although the flap was subsequently created by an automated microkeratome.

The next major innovation was the arrival on the scene in 2001 of the femtosecond laser to create the flap in LASIK, replacing the microkeratome (oscillating metal blade). IntraLase (the brand name of the first femtosecond laser to be approved in the US for the creation of the flap of corneal tissue in the first step in LASIK) became the new way to perform LASIK. The microkeratome was redundant; it was no longer necessary for a blade to touch the eye. This resulted in better safety, accuracy and clearer vision.

The most recent development in laser eye surgery was the development in 2008 of a new technique for treating short-sightedness and astigmatism called femtosecond lenticule extraction. In another application of the femtosecond laser, a thin, lens-shaped disc (or lenticule) was separated from the surrounding corneal tissue and then removed, resulting in the corneal shape required for clear unaided vision. This meant no corneal flap and no excimer laser. The procedure has further evolved to become SMILE laser, an acronym for small incision lenticule extraction. As the name suggests, the lenticule could now be extracted through a tiny laser-created key-hole incision in the cornea. SMILE was first introduced to Australia in 2012 and has found its place as a safe, accurate, and more modern procedure for correcting short-sightedness and astigmatism in many patients. The absence of a corneal flap means a less invasive procedure and less disturbance of corneal nerves compared to previous procedures. It is now emerging in the clinical data that SMILE laser may be a better choice for higher errors and drier eyes. ●

G.S

OTHER VISION CORRECTION PROCEDURES

Implantable Lenses

Implantable lenses (also called phakic intraocular lenses, where 'phakic' means that you retain your natural lens as distinct from replacing it) were first used in the 1980s in an attempt to correct very high spectacle prescriptions. Since then, designs have improved considerably and they have developed into a compelling option for a certain group of people who wear very uncomfortable, heavy glasses, or are struggling with contact lens wear and who are unsuitable for laser eye surgery on their cornea or lens. Implantable lenses can be used to correct very high amounts of short-sightedness or long-sightedness, especially in people under forty. Sometimes, implantable lenses are used when laser eye surgery is not an option due to the thickness or shape of your cornea, or if your glasses prescription is outside the normal range. The implantable lens is a tiny artificial lens designed to be placed permanently within your eye. One type sits between your cornea and iris, another type is placed behind the iris but in front of your natural lens. In both these cases your own natural lens remains untouched within your eye, providing that all-important ability to change focus between distance and near vision without effort in younger patients.

CASE STUDY

Here's a typical scenario. Maria, a very shy, quietly-spoken girl, aged twenty-four, presents for a vision correction consultation accompanied by her mother. Maria has worn very heavy glasses since she was a young girl. Even starting school at age 5, her glasses prescription was already -9 and since then her short-sightedness has increased so that she now wears a prescription of -16. Her mother tells me that Maria sometimes calls out to her at night because she can't find her glasses on her bedside table. Maria has tried contact lenses many times but is unable to manage them due to a dry eye condition as well as some chronic inflammation to her eyelids that makes contact lens wear very uncomfortable. So here we have a intelligent young woman who is completely dependent on a very heavy pair of glasses for absolutely everything. She can't go for a swim at the beach or the pool because she literally cannot see well enough to walk even a few meters without glasses. She has been for several laser vision correction consultations in the past and she has always been told that her glasses prescription is too high for the laser to correct. She and her mother now want to know if we could just laser as much as we can safely do and even reduce her glasses prescription so that she could wear a lighter, more attractive pair of glasses.

I examine her eyes. Her cornea is not particularly thick which means I can't treat more than about half of her glasses prescription with laser eye surgery. What she does have going for her though, is nice big eyes, so there is plenty of space inside her eye between the cornea and the iris and between the back of the iris and her lens. Maria is in fact an ideal candidate for an implantable lens. Laser eye surgery to her cornea is not going to address her problem as she will still need a strong pair of glasses even after surgery. Laser lens surgery could address all of her glasses prescription, but would rob her of her ability to change focus from distance to near – an ability that she will have for at least the next twenty years. However, an implantable lens would correct all of her prescription and preserve her own natural lens intact so that it can continue to provide focus at a range of distances for decades to come.

She can't go for a swim at the beach or the pool because she literally cannot see well enough to walk even a few metres without glasses.

Fig. 1

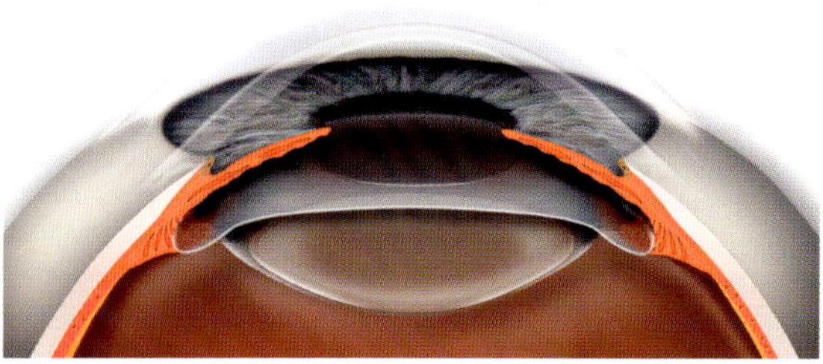

An implantable lens

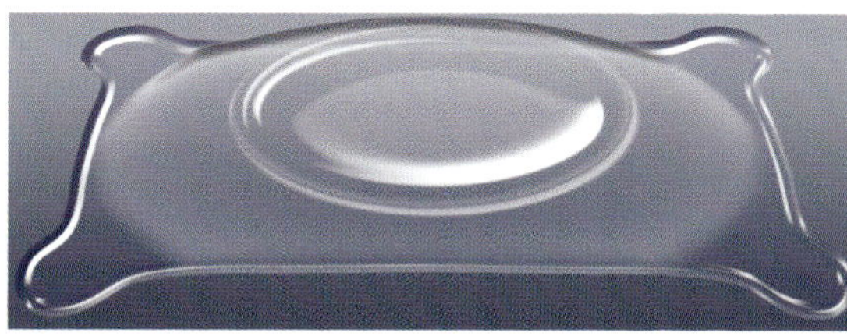

The implantable lens I recommend for her will sit in the space between her iris – the coloured part of her eye – and her natural lens *(Fig. 1)*. Another type of implantable lens actually 'clips' onto the iris but is invisible to the naked eye.

We talk about the benefits of surgery (which for her are very significant) and the risks (which, due to her good general health and the size of her eyes are relatively low) and she decides to have surgery. It goes very well and when she comes back for review a couple of months later, I finally see her smile for the first time. Her face lights up as she talks about her life without glasses. Days like those are what make my job so satisfying.

Why don't we just give implantable lenses to everyone, I hear you ask? Because, not everyone is a suitable candidate for these lenses. Implantable lens surgery is more involved than laser eye surgery and requires careful consideration of the benefits and risks before proceeding. LASIK or SMILE are always the procedures of choice for those who are suitable for it as it is so non-invasive, safe, predictable and effective. But not everyone is suitable for LASIK or SMILE.

When implantable lenses are placed in your eyes you cannot feel them at all. They require no maintenance and can achieve a good quality of vision. Also, they can be removed when, for example, you may require cataract surgery in the future. Your doctor will need to ensure that there is enough room inside the eye to allow fluid to flow properly around the implantable lens once it is placed in position. Once you have implantable lenses in place you will need an annual eye examination to make sure the lens maintains its correct position, that your intraocular pressure remains normal, that the cells on the back of the cornea are healthy, and that your natural lens remains clear.

Corneal Inlays

What are they, and are they any good? Corneal inlays are tiny donut-shaped discs or micro-lenses that are designed to sit within your cornea in a pocket created by a femtosecond laser. Typically, corneal inlays are only 3–4mm in size. Some inlays use the pinhole effect to improve near vision; the inlay is shaped like a small donut and the artificially small pupil it creates helps you to focus up close. Other designs build some power into a small thin lens that sits within the cornea. The procedure is minimally invasive and the inlays can be removed at a later date should another inlay be needed, or lens replacement surgery be required.

CASE STUDY

Here is a typical scenario. Chris, a well-spoken businessman, aged fifty two, comes to our practice to discuss vision correction. He is a builder by trade and runs a busy company which requires him to be on site as much as off. Chris jokes that he's had more pairs of reading glasses than most people have had dinners. They get lost, dusty, scratched, paint on them ... He has fabulous distance sight without glasses and doesn't want to compromise on that but would just like that little extra bit of reading vision so he can look at a blueprint or a packing slip on site. He also has a heavy vehicle license which requires him to have good distance vision in both eyes unless he wears glasses for driving. Some vision correction surgeons would offer someone like Chris a corneal inlay. This would involve the placement of a tiny ring within a specially created space in his cornea. The tiny donut-shaped ring would act a bit like a pinhole – not unlike those pinhole glasses you can get. The eye is in many ways like a camera and the pupil of our eye acts like the aperture of a camera – the smaller it is the better our focus becomes. Thus, when we try to read in poor light, our pupil dilates and it can be difficult to focus. If we read in bright sunlight, our pupil constricts right down and provides a pinhole to look through which makes our focus much sharper. That's why a good reading light makes such a difference! Not only does it provide better contrast making the print clearer, it also makes our pupil smaller and therefore, our focus sharper. So, in a similar way, a corneal inlay, in theory, can create an artificially smaller pupil and allow better focus up close.

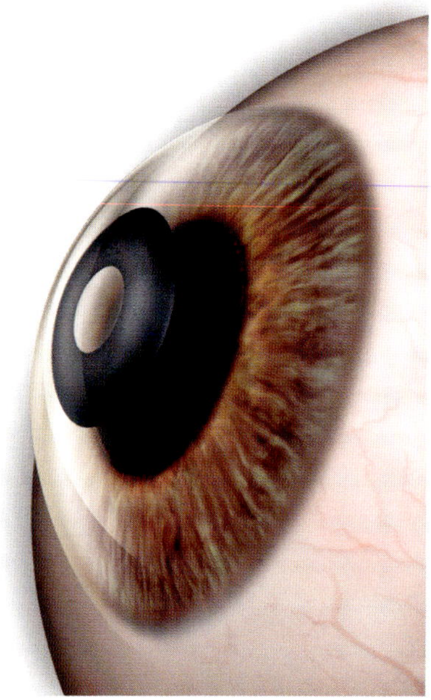

If we read in bright sunlight, our pupil constricts right down and provides a pinhole to look through which makes our focus much sharper. That's why a good reading light makes such a difference!

However, corneal inlays are one of the newest vision correction technologies and their effectiveness has yet to be fully established over time. Although interesting because they are potentially reversible, these technologies are, if anything, a fairly modest addition to the options available. Some patients will be happy, but a considerable minority takes a long time to achieve a good endpoint and some of the inlays will have to be removed. Careful patient selection is crucial. Simple blended vision achieved through LASIK or lens surgery (subject to a successful contact lens trial) is probably still a better alternative for the majority of patients who wish to decrease their dependence on reading glasses.

Are they any good? Well, the companies that make them think they are. The scientific theory is good and stacks up, but they are new. At this stage in the development of corneal inlays I wouldn't be recommending them to my friends or my patients. That may change in the future but I believe the future of vision correction surgery lies in improved lens replacement rather than inlays like this. Time will tell if I'm right. ●

M.L

DR RICHARD TROUTMAN

> *I am particularly proud of Dr Michael Lawless, who with my other Fellows has helped to carry José's "vision" to the world and who in 1991 pioneered Laser Vision Correction in Australia.*
>
> ***Dr Richard Troutman***

Dr Richard (Dick) Troutman is regarded by many as one the greatest corneal transplant surgeons of the twentieth century.

Along with other pioneering corneal surgeons such as Ramon Castroviejo, Townley Paton, Louis Paufique, Benjamin Rycroft, Joaquin Barraquer, Günter Mackensen and Heinrich Harms, he was highly innovative and very successful at taking ophthalmology to a completely new level. Troutman was instrumental in introducing the operating microscope to ophthalmology, which doesn't seem controversial, but it was very much so at the time in the 1950s and 1960s. There was great resistance from the profession to the use of operating microscopes because they were difficult to use and felt uncomfortable for surgeons who had never used them. But Troutman could see the enormous benefits of using them. His championing of the use of the operating microscope led to the development of many corneal procedures and he is now regarded as being the father of corneal microsurgery.

In the 1980s I was awarded a fellowship to work and study in New York under Dr Troutman at the Manhattan Eye, Ear and Throat Hospital. By then he was in his late sixties and had an international reputation as a corneal transplant expert. Having observed and assisted him in surgery, and operated under his instruction, I regard him as the greatest surgeon I have ever seen. The economy and precision in movement that he achieved was unparalleled and he was also inspirational in showing a young doctor like me how to lead a productive professional life.

Although Dick was based in New York all his professional life and was regarded as a pillar of corneal transplantation in the ophthalmology 'establishment', he had this interest in optics, vision correction surgery, and changing the shape of the cornea. All of this was seen as being just a little bit 'out there' at that stage. Dick was very open-minded about any new procedures and had an international view. For example, he knew both Fyodorov and Barraquer and the work they were doing. He was a close friend and colleague of both the Barraquer brothers (José in Bogota and Joaquin in Barcelona) and the first to understand and bring to the world what incredible things José Barraquer was doing. In fact, he sent me down to Colombia for a few months to work with José Barraquer.

When José Barraquer started reshaping the cornea through his keratomileusis technique to treat short-sightedness, Troutman understood how important this innovation was and then taught the procedure himself from his surgery in New York. This led to an understanding of what you could do to the corneal shape in order to correct short-sightedness and helped in understanding radial keratotomy and subsequently the PRK (ASLA) procedure. Troutman also used some of these ideas in treating corneal transplant astigmatism. He developed his own suture materials and suture types specifically for corneal transplant surgery. Dick Troutman was also a cautionary voice against the early intraocular lenses, which were sometimes released to market earlier than they should have been.

In 1982 Dick Troutman, José Barraquer and Miles Friedlander formed the International Society of Refractive Surgery as a vehicle for education for the entire profession in the burgeoning field of vision correction surgery. They realised that although Fyodorov was doing incredible things in Russia, and Barraquer was achieving significant break-throughs in Columbia, and Troutman was making ground-breaking advances in New York, the rest of the medical world didn't seem to know anything about it. José Barraquer was the first President of the Society of Refractive Surgery and Dick Troutman was the next President.

Dick Troutman has remained a firm friend. He is ninety years old and still attends the American Academy of Ophthalmology, and indeed he first attended when he was ten years old in 1932 because his father was an eye, ear, nose and throat surgeon at that stage when the specialties were combined. (He later specialised in ophthalmology only).

In 1991, after 46 years in the fascinating practice of ophthalmic microsurgery, just as the laser vision corrective techniques were ready for general clinical use, Dick retired from clinical practice. But his fertile imagination led him to design a particular chair for people with back pain, because he had suffered from back pain himself. The chair sales took off when it became known that the judge in the OJ Simpson trial was sitting on one of the Dick Troutman chairs. That murder trial was televised and played in front of the US public for almost year. There was comment at different times on the uniqueness of the judge's chair, so that was an unexpected situation where one of America's greatest doctors became famous for his chair design. ●

"It was my good fortune to know and work with Dr. José Barraquer, founder of the Clinica Barraquer de las Americas, in Bogota Columbia, for more than 30 years. In August 1966, just before the 20th International Congress of Ophthalmology in Munich, with Professors Günter Mackensen and Heinrich Harms, I founded the International Ophthalmic Microsurgery Study Group to which we invited over twenty international micro-surgeons with similar interests - among them José Barraquer – from around the world. It was at this and subsequent biennial meetings that José and I discovered and fostered our similar interests in vision correction surgery.

At the World Corneal Congress II in Washington DC in 1975, José entrusted me to introduce vision correction surgery to North America. In turn, in close cooperation with José, I began the training of a generation of my Corneal Fellows, each spending a part of their fellowship at the Clinica in Bogota under his personal supervision. I am particularly proud of Dr Michael Lawless, who with my other Fellows has helped to carry José's "vision" to the world and who in 1991 pioneered Laser Vision Correction in Australia. Internationally, recognised by his peers he is past President, 2001, of the International Society of Refractive Surgery with more than 3,000 members worldwide, and a past member of the editorial Board of The International Journal of Refractive Surgery, its highly respected monthly publication, (both of which I was responsible for founding). It is fitting that Dr Lawless should in turn co-author this volume with his own protégé and associate, Dr Gerard Sutton, the first Professor of Refractive Surgery in Australia and a pioneer of the new femtosecond laser for corneal transplant surgery."

Dr Richard Troutman

G.S

THE 13 MOST COMMON MYTHS ABOUT LASER VISION CORRECTION

The life so short, the craft so long to learn.
Hippocrates

Recently, I was asked at a lecture to speak about some of the common myths about laser eye surgery. I really had to think about that as I am working so closely with this technology and its incredible ability to correct vision, that it's easy to forget that laser eye surgery is still not well understood by the general public. Here are some of the most common myths I've encountered:

1 *You will never need to wear glasses again….*

The sad news for all of us is that your reading vision starts to go off, probably from your mid-forties. This is a universal fact. Our eyes have evolved over millions of years. The earliest complex eyes appear to have developed during the Cambrian Era, around 500 million years ago. And complex eyes evolved not once but dozens of times, in many different animals. But up until only a few hundred years ago – an evolutionary blink of an eye – life expectancy for humans was about 35–45 years. It was only when we started to live longer that we noticed these problems with our vision. Now that most of us live to at least seventy, or longer, we have to deal with this situation.

After the age of forty-five our natural lens within our eye becomes less elastic. It is therefore less able to change its shape to help us focus up close. So, if you've never worn glasses for distance and your distance vision is good, it will likely remain good, but you will need some extra help with focusing up close – for small print and things like that. Exercises won't help. And it degenerates with increasing age – whether you wear glasses or not – until by about fifty-seven years of age your lenses are rigid and cannot focus any nearer than about a metre.

So, even if you get laser vision correction to fix your short-sightedness in your twenties or thirties, most people will still need reading glasses when they reach middle age. All candidates for laser eye surgery are advised of this and, quite often, if they are nearing their mid-forties we deliberately leave one eye ever so slightly short-sighted so that eye can continue to read without reading glasses for longer.

A second group of people who may need to wear glasses again are those with very high glasses prescriptions – they may still end up slightly short-sighted after their laser vision correction. It is often possible to completely eradicate the need for glasses but not always and this is something that needs to be discussed before having a procedure as each individual case is different.

2 *The laser burns your eye...*

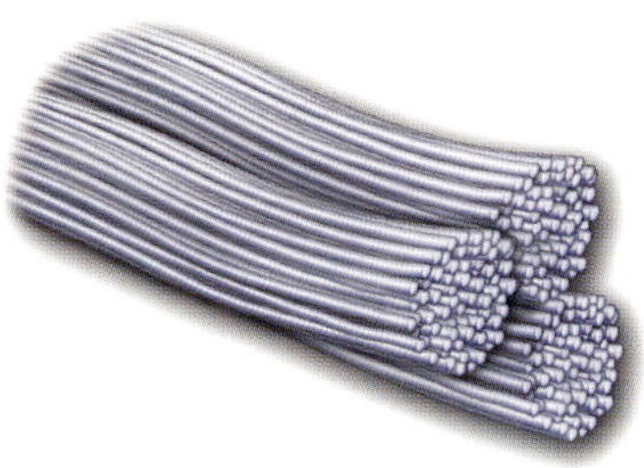

Absolutely not! Let's have another look at the structure of the cornea. Over 90% of it is made up of collagen, arranged into a thick layer called the stroma. The structure of collagen is very orderly. Each molecule is like a strand or micro-fibre. How these fibres are stacked (as well as the absence of any blood vessels) is what makes the cornea transparent. Imagine the collagen fibres stacked in neat rows and rows on top of each other, like a stack of drain-pipes on a building site.

They naturally fall into a very regular arrangement. This makes it possible for light waves to pass through the collagen fibres to the back of the eye. In a laser vision correction procedure, very specific parts of your corneal tissue are vaporised by the excimer laser. The way the laser works is it breaks the carbon bonds on the actual molecules within your cornea. **The laser does that through**

very fast pulses of energy without damaging or heating the surrounding tissues. The chemical reaction that occurs when the laser breaks these bonds raises the heat within the cornea to about 40 degrees Centigrade – about the same as a nice warm bath. But, as the laser's energy breaks the molecular bonds, it also causes the release of ozone (O_3) molecules into the surrounding air, which, if they make their way into your nostrils have that disconcerting smell reminiscent of sparks, or burning hair! However, most patients don't smell anything because this part of the procedure is very quick – it takes about 30 seconds – and the small amount of ozone released during the procedure is sucked up into a vacuum extractor. On rare occasions a patient may smell the ozone released and think, 'Oh my God, the laser's burning my eye!'

3 *We take out your eyeball to do the surgery…*

This one always brings a smile to my face! It reminds me of those entertainment console control systems on airplanes – the ones in the arm-rest of your seat where you pull it out and it's on a retractable cord so when you're finished you just give it a sharp yank and the whole thing slots back into place! Laser eye surgery is incredibly non-invasive. **Your eye stays firmly in your head at all times.** If you're having LASIK, all that happens is one laser works on your eye for fifteen seconds and a second laser works on it for about 30 seconds. Your eye is numbed with a single drop of local anaesthetic. There are two steps involved in LASIK. The first step involves creating a thin flap of corneal tissue. For this to happen, your eye's movements need to be stabilised so you feel some pressure on your eye as the stabilisation ring contacts your eye for about fifteen seconds while the femtosecond laser creates a tiny layer of microscopic bubbles just under the surface of your cornea. It's not painful. In the second step, the excimer laser removes tissue from very specific sites on the part of your cornea that is underneath the flap. You hear a tapping noise as the laser pulses and you see lights flashing. You may even get a faint whiff of ozone *(see myth 2. above)* but that's all. So, your eyeball never leaves your head. (Unless you donate it to science or medicine after your death! See *The Naked I*, page 154 for the story of the lost eye…*)*

4 *You can't have laser vision correction if you have astigmatism...*

Wrong. In the majority of cases, eyes with astigmatism can be treated with vision correction surgery. First I need to explain what astigmatism is. Most people hear the word at their optometrist's practice and unfortunately it is one of those words that sounds far worse than it actually is. 'Stigma' doesn't sound good, or people mix it up with 'strabismus', which is simply where the eyes are not looking in the same direction. Either way it sounds bad! But astigmatism is nothing sinister and is just a word to describe the shape of the cornea.

Astigmatism is something that most people just don't understand. And I'm not talking about the layman here. I would say probably nine out of ten medical students have no idea what astigmatism is so here's your chance! The eye is not made of precision-engineered steel; if this were the case they would all be perfectly shaped. No, the eye is a springy little rubber ball of a thing and even the fact that it is sitting in a socket in your skull can affect its shape. Your cornea is the clear dome-shaped window at the front of your eye. When you look at someone's eye, you look straight through it to the coloured iris beneath so it's easy to over-look it.

The clearly focused eye

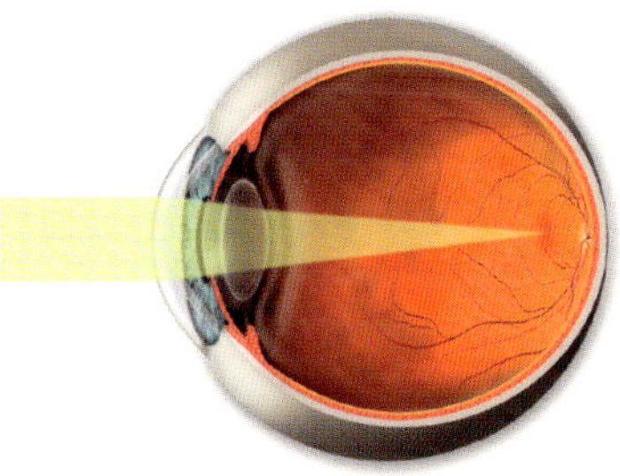

The cornea is responsible for bending light rays as they enter the eye so they focus clearly onto your retina. In order for the image on your retina to be clear, the cornea has to be exactly the right shape for your particular eye. If it's too curved, the image falls in front of the retina, too flat and the image falls behind the retina. But many corneas are slightly more curved in one direction than another. Imagine the cornea again like a dome. But this time it is more like a rugby ball shaped dome than a soccer ball shaped dome.

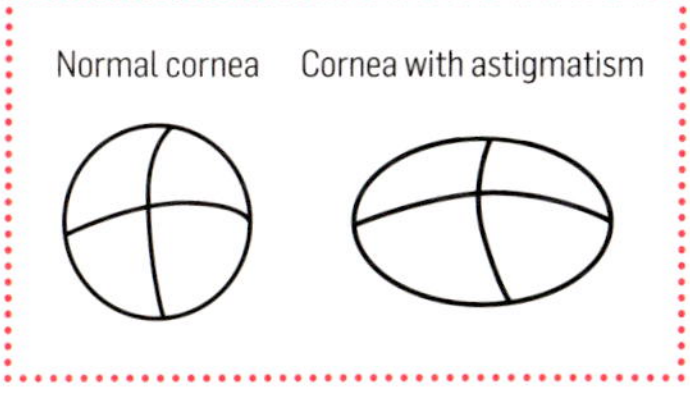

This is all astigmatism is – that slight difference between the two curves of the cornea. It's very common and completely normal. It results in some parts of the image falling closer to the retina than others, so some parts are more clearly in focus than others. It is actually more common to have a little bit of astigmatism than none at all so it is very normal. Most of the spectacles prescribed the world over contain a correction for at least a small amount of astigmatism. You now understand more about the shape of the cornea than nine out of ten med students!

Eyes with astigmatism can easily be treated with vision correction surgery in the majority of cases.

We simply remove more tissue from some parts of the cornea than others and that is part of the information that is programmed into the laser. Occasionally someone will have a very large degree of astigmatism and that causes all manner of problems – with glasses as well as contact lenses. In these cases the astigmatism is reduced but not always eliminated by a vision correction procedure.

5 *You can't have laser vision correction to get rid of reading glasses or multifocals...*

This is not true and I'm a perfect example of it. I have had laser vision correction surgery myself. It was performed by my colleague, Michael Lawless, a very safe pair of hands indeed. I think Michael has been one of the few Australian ophthalmologists who has achieved a genuine international reputation in refractive surgery. He is clearly one of the best refractive surgeons in Australia, if not in the world. I think he is a meticulous surgeon and a great craftsman in that regard. His attention to detail is his greatest strength, which is what you want in your surgeon.

At the time I was forty-six years old and struggling with my reading, but also seeing in the distance. One of the staff optometrists came in one day when I was working in my office. She had a patient file in her hand and she asked "What do you want to do about this patient?" As I pulled out my reading glasses she looked aghast and said "What do you think you are doing?"

"Oh, I'm getting a bit tired and old", I replied.

"You can't wear reading glasses," she shot back, "You're a laser eye surgeon." When I began to make excuses she said, "Gerard, at some stage you are going to have to eat your own dog food."

"You can't wear reading glasses," she shot back, "You're a laser eye surgeon. At some stage you are going to have to eat your own dog food."

It was a point well made, so I had a contact lens trial, just like film director, Bruce Beresford did (see *The Beauty of Blended Vision*, page 82). After the trial I asked Michael Lawless if he would operate on my eyes. I thought the result was fabulous. It doesn't keep me out of glasses for everything but I don't need glasses for distance, for working on the computer, or for looking at patients' notes. Occasionally I wear a pair of reading glasses at night-time. Another partner here, Dr Chris Rogers, did Michael's laser eye surgery and I operated on Dr Colin Chan, one of the other laser eye surgeons at our practice. So we do eat our own dog food.

6 *Once you have laser surgery you can't have it again…*

Yes. You can. **Occasionally we also need to do an enhancement procedure because of a small amount of residual error.** My enhancement rate is about 1–2%. And it is usually a fairly straightforward procedure. I re-lift the flap, the laser removes a tiny amount of corneal tissue to fine-tune the result and then I put the flap back.

Most people who I agree to operate on get a result that they are very happy with. I would say that the satisfaction rate with my patients is over 98%. That is in part due to a very careful selection process. At least 20% of the people that come to me for laser vision correction don't end up having it. We talk them out of it. Maybe their cornea is too thin or an unusual shape, or their glasses prescription too high, or, their tear quality isn't good enough (*see myth 9. below*) or, their expectations are simply not realistic.

7 *The laser does the procedure automatically. You don't need a surgeon – anyone could do it.*

This is of course completely untrue. The best example I can think of is NASA's space program; although their space shuttles are highly computerised, the astronauts need a vast amount of training to stay on top of every conceivable situation. Complex eye surgery is no different and the path to becoming an ophthalmologist is a long one. You start with a basic degree in medicine, which can take six or seven years to complete. Then you have to complete three years of general doctor training in a hospital as an intern and a resident. After that you make a decision about whether you are going to become a General Practitioner or a specialist. If you want to do ophthalmology you must sit a very tough exam and if you get through you then have to complete another four years training – ophthalmologist specialist surgical training. At the end of that you can go out and practice if you wish, but if you want to be a *sub-specialist* – or have a special area of expertise – then you have to do a fellowship, which takes between one and three years. I did my fellowship with Michael Lawless and Chris Rogers and then went overseas for a further two years to do specialist training in England and Germany as laser vision correction was such a new area.

No matter how advanced the technology, an expert surgeon needs to drive the entire procedure and manage the variability of responses.

Because vision correction surgery is a relatively new field of medicine, there was, for a long time, no formal training place for it anywhere in the world. The refractive surgery degree at Sydney University was set up because there were a lot of doctors who were finishing their ophthalmology training at the end of four years and then just going out and doing laser eye surgery without adequate training. I was pleased to be involved in setting up the course in refractive (vision correction) surgery at Sydney University in order to address that need. When doctors finished their ophthalmology training they could do a further twelve month course and be competent in doing vision correction surgery. As an Examiner at the college, the other thing I was involved in was providing more tuition to the registrars during their training, which did not exist previously because up until about five years ago, vision correction surgery was seen as being outside mainstream ophthalmology.

The long and the short of it is this; no matter how advanced the technology, an expert surgeon needs to drive the entire procedure and manage the variability of responses.

8 *Laser vision correction is risky... lots of things can go wrong.*

Laser vision correction is the safest and most successful procedure in modern medicine. I'm not taking any chances with my own eyes or my patients' eyes. Because we have been performing these procedures for decades on thousands of patients we have evidence which clearly shows that laser vision correction is very safe. The risk of a major complication is less than 0.02% (or one in five thousand). That can still worry some people but to put it into perspective, the estimated risk of a sight-threatening complication from soft contact lens wear is about 0.006% (or one in 16,000) per year.[5]

By far the most common complications after laser vision correction – both corneal and lens surgery – are

- a residual error, meaning that not all of your glasses prescription was eliminated by the surgery and
- dry eye, which in the vast majority of cases where patient selection has been rigorous, is temporary.

We've never had an infection from laser eye surgery at our practice. In the fifteen years that I have practiced there, day in day out, with many of the same staff throughout all those years, I have never seen a laser eye surgery disaster.

Our patients often show their appreciation for our work. I've had one patient send me a dozen red roses, which is fine, but it's an unusual reaction, especially as it was a guy! I keep all of the thank you cards that people give me so I have a folder full of thank you cards because

I like that. When people are trusting their eyes to us then we need to be delivering for them. Obviously as a professional you want to be doing the best than you can for the patient, but when you get a thank you card on top of that, a heartfelt thank you saying that laser eye surgery has changed people's lives, then that is extremely satisfying. I believe ours is a unique environment, with highly skilled surgeons – several of whom have international reputations – supported by a professionally trained staff. Perhaps it is a positive reflection on our work practices that the staff are so loyal. They are like part of my extended family. We have all been on this remarkable journey together.

Even so, there will always be a sector of society who wear glasses or contact lenses, often unhappily, but would never consider laser eye surgery because they have concerns about the risks, no matter how small they really are.

9 *Laser vision correction causes dry eyes…*

This can happen, but if it does it's usually temporary. Tears; why do we need them? Our tears are under-estimated. Most people think of them as just water. But they are so much more! Our tear film is actually made up of three layers.

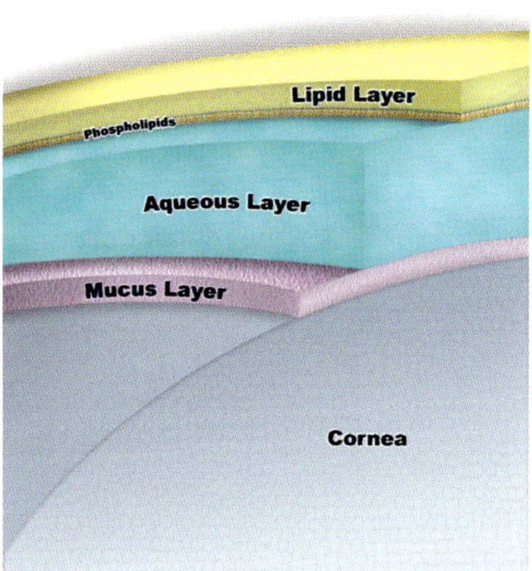

The central layer – or aqueous layer – is by far the thickest and consists mainly of water. These tears are produced in your lacrimal gland, located above the eye (behind your eyebrow), and they are the ones which run like crazy when we cut an onion or watch a sad movie. The aqueous layer also has lots of antibodies in it, which I'll come back to. On top of that watery layer is an oily layer and this oil is produced in a row of tiny glands which run along the inside edge of each eyelid. They are constantly squeezing tiny amounts of oil into your tear film which prevent it

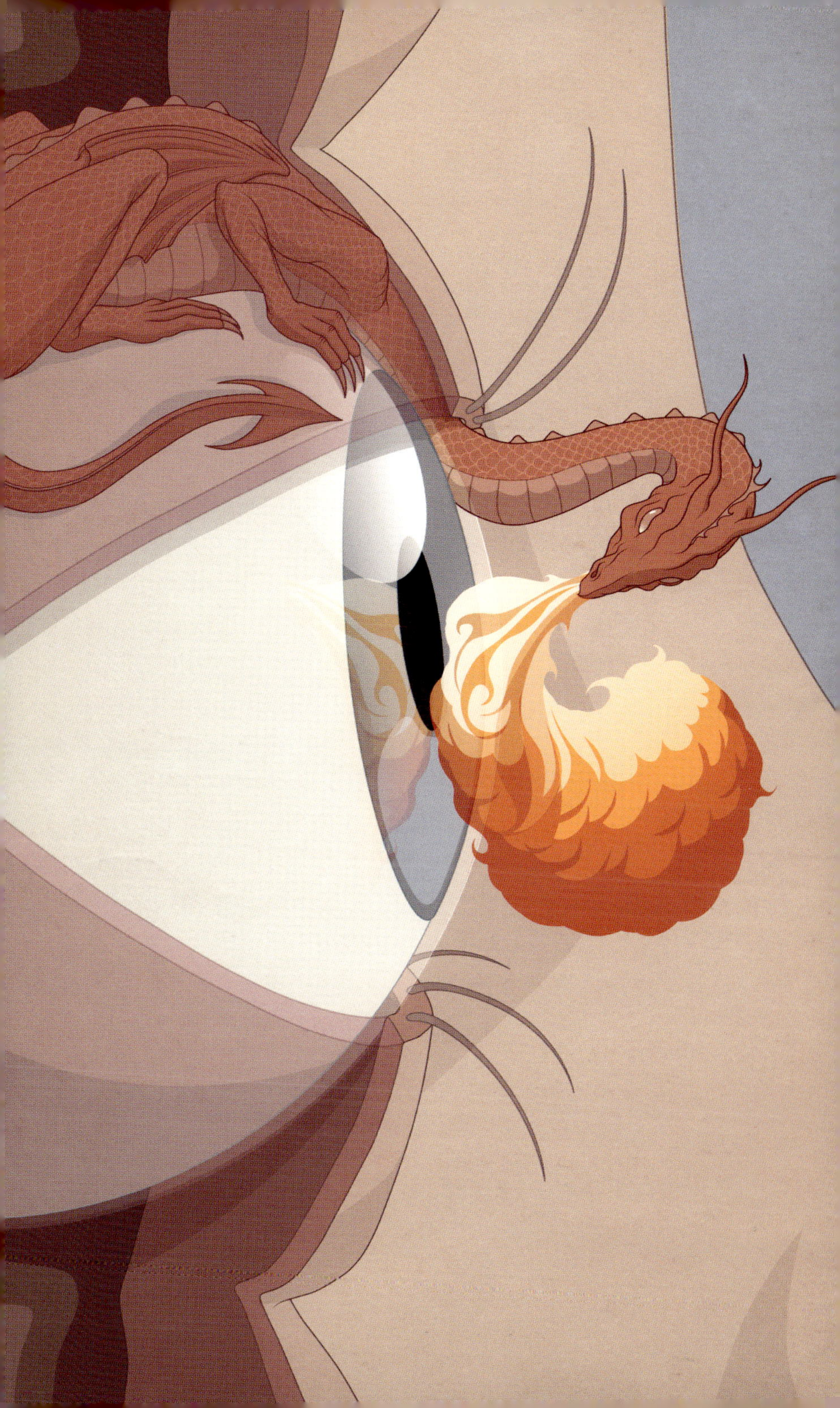

evaporating. The third layer is a thin layer of mucus which helps stick your tear layer onto your eye and spread out over the eye and coat it nicely. The corneal surface has a coating of tiny finger-like structures – like Velcro – and the mucus acts like the other half of the Velcro and attaches the tear layer firmly on.

The surface of the eye is an almost sterile environment. Unlike our mouth which typically contains about 20 billion microbes, the surface of our eye has virtually none! Individual bacteria are always falling into our eye off our lids and lashes and they quickly get swept away by the blinking action of the lids and gobbled up by the antibodies in the tear film. Our tear film protects our cornea from infection and from drying out. If it dries out it is no longer smooth and shiny and not only does it feel sore, but we can't see properly. It's a bit like trying to see through your windscreen when it's coated with a film of dirt; you need to switch on the wipers (blink) and squirt some water (tears) to get it clear again. Our cornea needs to stay moist and lubricated to be healthy and it has lots of tiny nerve endings that cry out in discomfort if the tear film doesn't do its job well. This triggers our lacrimal gland to produce more of our watery (or reflex) tears. So, our tear film is essential for clear vision as well as helping our eyes feel good.

What happens to our tear film after we have laser vision correction? When the flap is created during LASIK, it disturbs some of the corneal nerves. Does this mean its hurts? No, quite the opposite actually, and therein lies the problem. During the procedure itself the cornea is anaesthetised but afterwards, once the effect of the drops wears off, the cornea is *less* sensitive than usual so it doesn't actually produce as many aqueous tears as usual. This results in the tear film drying out a bit and the underlying cornea drying out too, leading to fluctuating clarity of vision. As the corneal nerves regenerate in the early weeks and months after the LASIK procedure, the corneal sensitivity returns to normal and so does the tear production. **Dry eye is by far the most common side effect we see after LASIK and it affects most people. It is usually temporary and easily managed with the artificial tear drops provided. Patients with chronic or severe dry eye problems require careful consideration and are often unsuitable for LASIK in particular. SMILE laser and ASLA have a lesser effect on corneal nerves and are more appropriate procedures for those with drier eyes.**

(10) *They cut your eye with a blade during laser vision correction*

Not any more they don't. Up until October 2004, LASIK was not an all-laser procedure. As you now know, the LASIK procedure involves two steps. In the first, a flap is created and in the second, the underlying cornea is re-shaped with a laser. At our practice and indeed most practices in Australia, these two steps are now done using two different lasers. The femtosecond laser is used to create the flap and the excimer laser reshapes the cornea. However, the femtosecond laser has only been available in Australia since 2004. Prior to that, the flap in LASIK was created using an oscillating metal blade called a microkeratome.

The microkeratome was used to create the flap in LASIK until 2004.

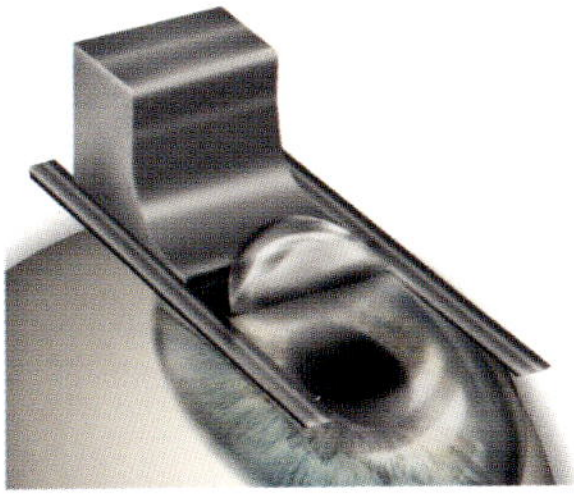

The femtosecond laser now creates the corneal flap.

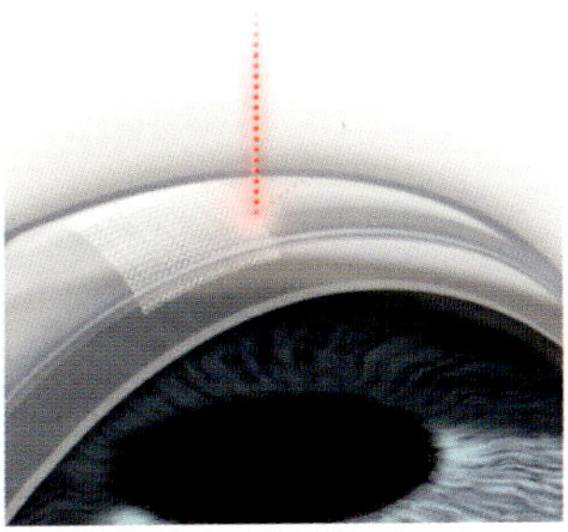

(11) *Laser eye surgery is scary...*

It may sound scary, but it doesn't need to be. It is very normal to be scared of any surgical intervention on the eye. Even though laser vision correction is the safest, most predictable procedure in modern medicine, it still ranks as one of the scariest things that you may contemplate in your life. Back in the 1990s a US study found it rated as the 3rd most stressful event in your life … and only after death and marriage! Why *are* people afraid of laser eye surgery? Is it to do with the eyes? We're all a bit funny about our eyes. I know I am. People think it's just them. They say, "You don't know me doctor, I'm a bit funny about anything near my eyes." That is something I hear all the time.

Is it to do with lasers maybe? The idea in popular culture of a laser as a lethal weapon… I've had a patient sitting in the examination room with her 10 month old playing with a Buzz Lightyear plastic toy on the floor and as we are discussing a possible vision correction plan all I can hear is Buzz's inimitable voice urging "I have a laser and I will use it"!

Laser eye surgery has had a short and at times turbulent history. There have been plenty of procedures performed with less than ideal outcomes and it is only in the past 10 years that we have really been able to address all the safety issues completely. In terms of outcomes, laser eye surgery is now one of the safest procedures in modern medicine.

12 *You can see better after laser eye surgery than you could with your glasses…*

This isn't really a myth. It doesn't happen all the time but it does happen quite often. The laser reshapes your cornea to a slightly better shape for sharp vision to occur compared to the shape of your glasses lenses. Occasionally, and this is certainly not something we promote because it doesn't always happen, but sometimes you will get someone who can see a whole extra line on the vision chart compared to when they had their glasses or contact lenses. This is because the laser reshapes the cornea to a technically very advanced shape. It's even better than nature, God forbid!

An adult with perfect vision can read the small letters of the eye-test chart at six metres (or twenty feet, as in 20/20 vision). These letters are very small – right at the limit of what human eyes can see – and are roughly a little under a centimetre in height. Not all species are the same. 20/20 vision is usually the best level of vision for humans. But a wedge tail eagle can see the same letter at *five times* that distance – so from one hundred feet they can see that letter. The eagle just has a different kind of eye and a different way that it is hardwired to their brain.

So, can you see better than 20/20 after laser eye surgery? It is true, and not just at our practice, that many patients who have laser vision correction report seeing better than they ever have in their lives.

Here's an extract from a letter from a patient who happened to be a pilot in the Royal Australian Air Force:

"When I had my laser eye surgery I no longer needed my distance vision glasses. But something else also happened. My vision became much sharper and I could see things that I had never been able to see before in my life, even in my glasses. Individual leaves on trees in the distance, the tiny LEDs that make up the circle of red light on a traffic light. And when I have my eyes tested now I can read far better than 20/20 vision. I can now read

those letters at twice the distance that I could see before. What does this mean for me? Well, it actually means life or death. As a pilot in the Royal Australian Air Force I can now see a plane or missile approaching from twice the distance I could see it before. It is a serious advantage."

Believe it or not, a number of pilots from the Kuwait Air Force came to see us. It is not a particularly big Air Force but they sent their pilots all the way from Kuwait to come and have surgery with us as they wanted to get out of glasses. That was interesting because they all flew out, had the surgery, and then they flew back again and their last correspondence indicated that they were all going well. Both Michael and I consult for the armed forces, so we saw a lot of the SAS guys before they were deployed in Iraq and Afghanistan. We knew there was something coming on because they sent their SAS soldiers who wore glasses or contact lenses to have their surgery done before they were deployed. That mixes it up a bit. They are not your average run of the mill type of patient.

And lastly, just for fun....

13 *If you have laser vision correction you will have more sex....*

Ah yes, this is my all-time favourite myth. This myth is definitely not based on any clinical findings that I've ever seen – unfortunately – but it is certainly true that laser vision correction can change your life in all sorts of unexpected ways. A happy patient described how she felt about not needing glasses anymore ... *"The other thing that was really life-changing was that I took all my glasses up to OPSM and handed them over. If you hand them over they send them overseas to a charity. I had a huge big David Jones bag of glasses. I know them up at OPSM really well because my little boy wears glasses and we are up there just about every second week because he breaks them at school and we are getting them repaired. So I am there giving my sack of glasses to them and saying how I don't need them anymore. It was really quite liberating handing over all these pairs of glasses but it also felt quite weird. It was great!"*

So, while it's unlikely that laser vision correction will improve your love life, it often changes the way people feel about themselves. ●

M.L

DR MARGUERITE MCDONALD

One of the recognised pioneers of laser vision correction is Marguerite McDonald. She blazed the trail for women in ophthalmology by being a great clinician, a dedicated scientist and a terrific role model.

Marguerite was a resident in ophthalmology at the Manhattan Eye, Ear and Throat Hospital, and in the 1980s went on to do a fellowship in cornea at Louisiana State University (LSU). Marguerite performed the first excimer laser procedure in the world on a normal short-sighted person in New Orleans in 1988.

Much of her research at Louisiana State University took place in a small room on campus where, as it happened, there was a lot of building work going on. This coincidence proved to have serendipitous benefits to our understanding of laser eye surgery. In the 1980s, when the excimer laser was first used on the cornea, it would give very discrete tissue removal, i.e. it removed specific portions of corneal tissue and left adjacent areas untouched. The problem was it was too precise! What wasn't known at the time was that the edges of the zones where the laser was removing tissue needed to be smooth to avoid scarring or haziness developing in the clear cornea. However, at Marguerite's surgery, because there was a lot of vibration around because of the building work being carried out, the constant vibration actually made the laser "jitter" which resulted in little overlapping areas of tissue removal. Marguerite realised that this actually led to better outcomes and an improvement in the technique whereby a smoothing effect was applied to give a better transition zone between treated and untreated cornea. Naturally, she had been complaining loudly and vigorously about the inconvenience of the building work, trying to get it stopped. Thankfully, the university administrators took no notice of her and she began to achieve consistently beneficial outcomes for her patients which led to a new understanding of how to make the best use of the excimer laser.

As well as being an outstanding ophthalmologist, Marguerite was also a great storyteller. Many years ago she was a spectator at the US Open at Flushing Meadow, sitting in the crowd. The man seated on one side of her was a short, but very solid person who spoke with a thick Austrian accent. He struck up a conversation with the beautiful, well-spoken woman seated on the other side of Marguerite. They kept talking across her and it was abundantly clear to Marguerite that the Austrian man and the American woman were hitting it off. In the end Marguerite stood up and offered to move seats so that they could sit together. When she later saw photographs in the newspaper of the blossoming romance and subsequent marriage of Arnold Schwarzenegger and Maria Shriver, Marguerite realised they were the couple who had met while sitting either side of her at the US Open. She feels partly responsible for that couple getting together.

In 2001 Marguerite served as President of the American Society of Cataract and Refractive Surgery, which was the same year that I was President of the International Society of Refractive Surgery, so we had a lot to do with each other. She is still in practice, but after hurricane Katrina, relocated to New York and is now practising in upstate New York. ●

G.S

PROFESSOR JOHN MARSHALL

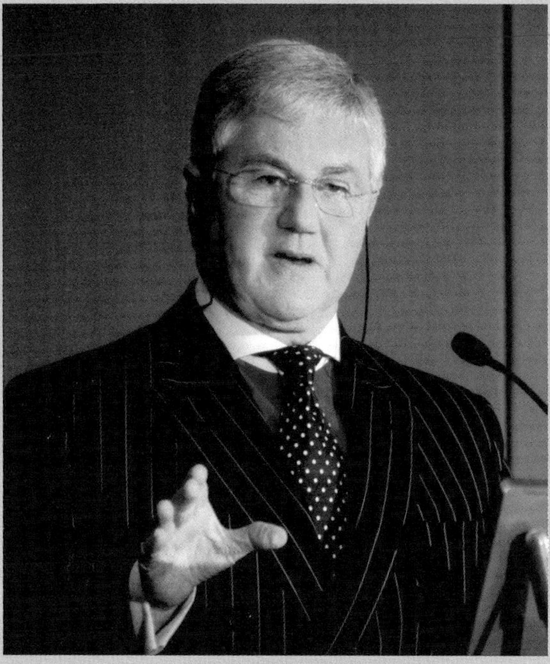

Professor John Marshall giving a lecture in Athens

No book covering the history of eye surgery would ever be complete if mention was not made of Professor John Marshall.

Currently, he is Emeritus Professor of Ophthalmology at Kings College, London and also Professor of Ophthalmology at the Institute of Ophthalmology in association with Moorfield's Eye Hospital and one of the most sought-after speakers in the world on all forms of laser. He has won a swag of international awards for his work in ophthalmology.

In the mid-1980s John Marshall conceptualised the idea of 'laser ablation' with the excimer laser and was awarded a patent on the technique. Up until then, others were focused on replicating radial keratotomy with the excimer laser instead of with a blade. The excimer laser was being used to create radial excisions in the peripheral parts of the cornea. But Marshall understood that the key lay in sculpting a whole area of the cornea with the excimer laser and not just discrete areas. His concept of the lenticular cut, i.e. where a central disc of tissue is removed rather than radial cuts, completely changed the way laser eye surgery was performed.

Over the past forty years John Marshall has conducted research which focused on the inter-relationship between light and ageing and the development of lasers for use in ophthalmic diagnosis and surgery and he has published over a thousand papers. As well as inventing many 'laser' techniques and applications, John is also an expert in the user of lasers in the military and how they can affect the eyes.

Back in 1995 I worked as his research fellow and not long after I started, he kindly invited my wife and me to a barbecue at his 'house' in Wimbledon. Not forgetting my manners, I recall asking him if it was a casual affair and if so, would **thongs** be appropriate ... Thongs of course are practically a compulsory item of footwear for Australian barbecues, but the English don't call them that; they go by the name of 'flip-flops' over there. Thongs on the other hand mean something quite different (and rather more risqué) to the English ... I think everyone was most relieved when I arrived wearing a pair of shorts and the afore-mentioned footwear! John was a terrific host, quick with his charismatic smile and, like myself, quite fond of a good Burgundy. ●

CONCLUSION: THEY CAME, THEY SAW, THEY CONQUERED

The first fossils of eyes that have been found thus far date from about 540 million years ago and since that time the eye has evolved into the most astonishing part of the human anatomy. What we see, what we experience, even what we turn a blind eye to, dominates so much of our everyday lives. And yet, in that context, the history of vision correction by surgical means has barely begun. Dr Tsutomu Sato carried out the first form of vision correction surgery in the 1930s. It was then a radical experimental procedure, which it remained for many decades, as visionaries like Ridley, Fyodorov and Barraquer worked tirelessly to unlock the secrets to successfully improving the vision of their patients through surgical intervention.

Isaac Newton, the English physicist, mathematician and astronomer famously said, "If I have seen further, it is by standing on the shoulders of giants." And so it is with us. In our own humble way we have followed in the footsteps of our 'giants', Sato, Ridley, Fyodorov and Barraquer. If they were alive today we believe they would be delighted to see the amazing developments brought about by the surgery they pioneered and would be very proud of the results we are able to achieve for our patients.

We began working in ophthalmology as young men and in the course of our professional careers have seen the most profound changes in laser vision correction surgery. It is no longer experimental, but now commonplace, accurate in terms of outcomes and, most importantly, safe. The advances, particularly in the last five years with femtosecond laser lens surgery, have resulted in procedures which are light-years ahead of where it all began less than eighty years ago. Ophthalmology is proud of its scientific traditions and we see ourselves as being custodians of that knowledge and using the skills we have developed as surgeons to do everything we can to improve the vision of our patients.

We trust that you, the reader, whether you are a prospective patient, or scientist, or optometrist, or colleague have found our book informative, enjoyable and enlightening. Both of us believe that what we do is incredibly special, and even after careers of many decades we still get a thrill at being able to give some of our patients clarity of vision for the first time in their lives. And yet in so many ways all we are doing is giving nature a helping hand so that people can see the beauty that surrounds them, or as was so aptly put by the late great Louis Armstrong:

The colors of the rainbow, so pretty in the sky
Are also on the faces of people going by,
I see friends shaking hands,
Saying, 'How do you do?'
They're really saying, 'I love you'.

PROCEDURES IN A NUTSHELL

	LASIK	ASLA (Advanced Surface Laser)
Age	20+ (subject to a stable spectacle prescription)	20+ (subject to a stable spectacle prescription)
Prescription Range	+4 to -10	+3 to -8
Visual Recovery	Very quick visual recovery – usually over-night	Visual recovery slower than LASIK – at least a week of down-time recommended
Discomfort	Very little discomfort during healing	Range of discomfort during early days of healing ranges from mild to moderate
Price Range	Mid to higher price range	Mid to higher price range
Safety Profile	Excellent safety profile	Excellent safety profile
Suitability	Not suited to thin or steep corneas or chronic dry eyes	Procedure of choice for thinner (healthy) corneas and some dry eye conditions
Level of Invasiveness	Relatively non-invasive – only involves cornea	Relatively non-invasive – only involves cornea
Other	Can cause temporary dry eye	

SMILE Laser	Laser Lens Surgery (Clear Lens Replacement)	Laser Cataract Surgery	Implantable Lenses
20+ (subject to a stable prescription)	50+	50+	22 to 50
Currently -3 to -10 (including astigmatism)	Caters for a very wide range of spectacle prescriptions	Caters for a very wide range of spectacle prescriptions	Caters for a very wide range of spectacle prescriptions
Very quick – within a few days	1–2 days	1–2 days	1–2 days
Very little discomfort during healing	Minimal. Often foreign body sensation overnight	Minimal. Often foreign body sensation overnight	Minimal. Often foreign body sensation overnight
Mid to higher price range	Higher price range	Higher price range	Higher price range
Excellent safety profile	Excellent safety profile	Excellent safety profile	Excellent safety profile established in suitable candidates
More suited than LASIK to higher errors and drier eyes	Care in high myopia	Only in presence of clinically significant lens opacity	Healthy cornea and roomy eye required
Relatively non-invasive, corneal involvement only	Relatively more invasive than a corneal procedure	Relatively more invasive than a corneal procedure	Relatively more invasive than a corneal procedure
		Rebate from Medicare and health fund if applicable	

You are not here merely to make a living.
You are here in order to enable the world
to live more amply, with greater vision,
with a finer spirit of hope and achievement.
You are here to enrich the world, and you
impoverish yourself if you forget the errand.

Woodrow Wilson

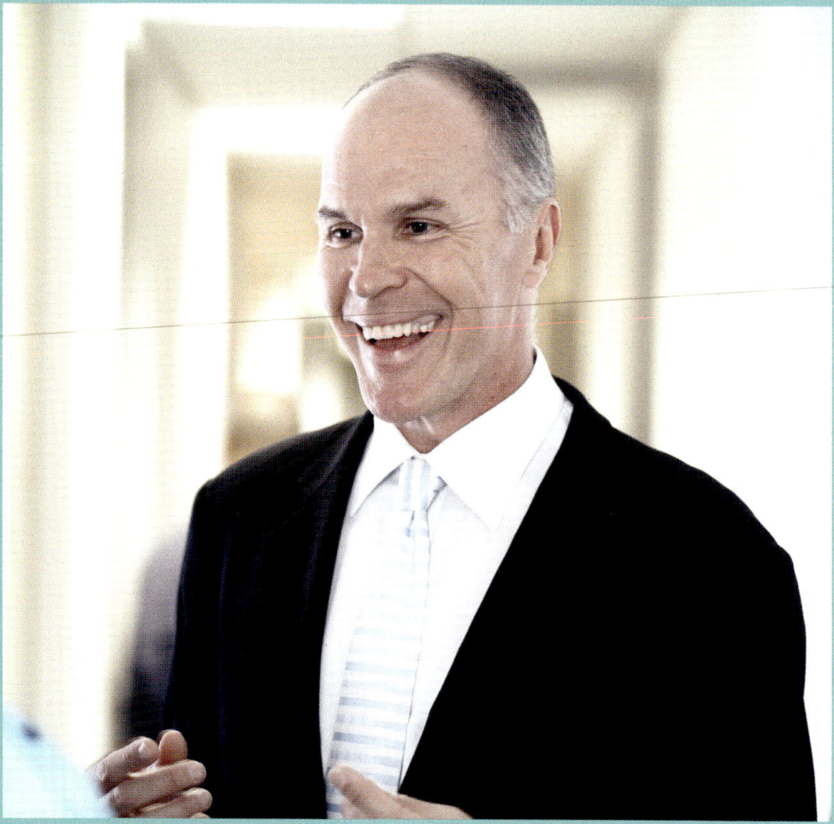

THE NAKED I
MICHAEL LAWLESS

Tell us something about you that very few people know.
At the age of twelve I sang a semi-religious song called *The Legend* and won the boy soprano solo section of the City of Sydney Eisteddfod.

If they made a movie of your life, who would be the best Hollywood actor to play you?
Clint Eastwood, without a doubt. I first saw him when I watched far too much daytime TV as a young boy in the late 1960s and Clint was the star of the series *Rawhide*. This was before he became famous for things like *Dirty Harry*, but even then he portrayed that terrific sense of calm and capable self-assurance that is so admirable.

What is the worst piece of advice you were ever given?
When I was in the Navy I was wondering whether I should consider a career in ophthalmology. Then we had a visit by a very experienced physician from Melbourne and I asked him what he thought of my idea. "Don't do it," he replied. "The exams are too difficult and you'll never get in." He had me pegged as a navy doctor – nothing more – nothing less – and in hindsight it was terrible advice. Ophthalmology was perfectly suited to me.

And I know it wasn't the question but the best piece of advice I was given, and I mean professional advice, was by ophthalmologist and friend Dick Troutman. When I first started out doing laser vision correction back in 1991, Dick Troutman said to me "Look, it might be a great career you are going to have, but the problem is that you are going to get too busy.

Take *a day a week* away from work and *think* about things, research things and write things. Collect your data, analyse them and write about them. It might seem that you would be better off doing something else – and you will certainly make more money by doing something else – but follow my advice, and that way you will continue to have credibility and more and more authority within the profession, and also it will be more interesting as you will acquire all this knowledge and it will make your practice-life very interesting."

I've always been a Churchillophile. I love the way he writes and thinks. I admire his bravery against all the odds and the way he lived his life.

So I did that and my partners Chris Rogers and Peter Cohen embraced that as well, as did Gerard Sutton when he came on board a couple of years later. We published the first paper on laser vision correction in Australia in *Modern Medicine* in 1992 and the following year we published our clinical results in the *Medical Journal of Australia.* Then we went on to publish and publish, and we now have, between Gerard and I, hundreds of publications in the peer-reviewed literature and text book chapters. All this data from thousands and thousands of procedures – we collected it, analysed it and the process has become more and more sophisticated. It has reached the stage today where we have a full-time researcher who is skilled in biostatistics. In the early days it was primitive. We were just learning it all. Now it is a well-oiled machine of data collection, analysis and reporting. It has continued for twenty five years.

What is your idea of perfect happiness?
I believe that 'perfect' is the enemy of good. There is no such thing as perfect happiness. You need to be content with things in your life and that leads to happiness.

What is your earliest memory?
In hospital getting my tonsils out. I must have been about four years old. Someone gave me a bottle of Coca Cola which I had never had before. Obviously, it was a real treat. I reached up and knocked it over and it spilled all over the floor. It is such a vivid memory – I can still the bottle falling – see my desperate attempt to stop it – and then this black liquid covering the hospital floor. What a sad little boy I was that day.

Is there a person, or a book or film or an event that changed your life?
Meeting my wife Alison, no question about it. I was invited to a dinner party one Saturday night which I was quietly dreading as I was quite a shy person and knew most of the guests would be complete strangers. I had had a few drinks before I arrived which I figured would get me through the evening. When I walked in Alison was there sitting at the table. She was a last minute addition to the guest list. I thought she was fantastic and I still do.

What was the most embarrassing thing that happened to you when you were growing up?
For some unknown reason I was a great blusher as a youth. I blush even thinking about it now. It's find myself in a social situation going red for no good reason and then when I realised I was blushing I would be even more embarrassed.

What do you consider the most overrated virtue, and why?
Chastity. It's a virtue encouraged or imposed by many different religions for no discernible benefit other than to make the vast majority of people feel a sense of shame or embarrassment for doing something everyone agrees is perfectly natural.

If you could invite five people from history to a barbecue at your place, who would they be and why?
These would be my guests and in this order: First, Genghis Khan. I'd like to hear how such a horrible person could control half the world. You'd have to anticipate that he'd be trouble as a guest. Second, Winston Churchill. I've always been a Churchillophile. I love the way he writes and thinks. I admire his bravery against all the odds and the way he lived his life. My third guest would have to be Jesus and accompanying him I would have Mohammed. Imagine having the opportunity of talking to the pair of them. And my last guest would be my Dad. I would have my Dad back so that he could meet them all as well.

What is your most treasured possession?
My father's wedding ring. When I was a little kid I used to hold his hand and feel this huge gold band on his finger. It's engraved with the date that he married Mum – 1948 – and when he was dying he gave it to me. It reminds me of him.

Tell us something about your co-author, Dr Sutton, that most people don't know.

I've known Gerard for twenty years and worked closely with him during this time, almost on a daily basis. Like a lot of specialists, including myself, Gerard went overseas for further training and worked at Moorfields Eye Hospital and St Thomas's in London. The training is almost priceless, and they pay you a pittance. Gerard, his wife, and their two very young children were living in what was then one of the most expensive cities in the world with not a lot of money to go around. One way to save money was to avoid catching the tube and walking to work. In his last few months there, Gerard developed a hole in his only pair of shoes. As he simply couldn't afford a new pair, he grabbed one of the kid's packs of cards and put a card over the hole each day before he set off to the hospital. Then when it started to snow Gerard began arriving at work with wet socks. His boss heard this squelching sound as he walked past and asked what was going on. He showed her the hole and explained the situation. "How long have you been walking to work with a hole in your shoe?" she asked.

His boss heard this squelching sound as he walked past and asked what was going on. He showed her the hole and explained the situation. "How long have you been walking to work with a hole in your shoe?"

"A couple of months."

As the British are such sticklers on things like dress, Gerard half expected her to admonish him for not wearing clothing appropriate for a doctor. Instead, she asked Gerard if she could have his shoes when his time was up and he moved back to Australia. "Why?" he wanted to know.

"Because, I'm going to have them framed," she announced. "I want to show others studying in this hospital what is required to succeed here." When he left he duly handed over the shoes and by all accounts they were framed and hung in her office.

Gerard's timing was perfect. He came back to Australia at the very time when there was enormous public interest in laser eye surgery. Everyone wanted to have it done, but there was a severe shortage of surgeons who were capable of doing it. I've come across plenty of good surgeons, but to me he is in a class of his own. Technically, he is excellent. He makes good decisions and deals with issues when they arise, but doesn't squib the difficult things. Gerard is meticulous and never leaves a thing undone. He is exactly what you want as a patient, because you will be looked after, and looked after by an expert.

My favourite gadget is...
The femtosecond laser machine which I use for cataract and laser lens surgery. I have had a lot of great gadgets over twenty-five years, but it is just magical.

I wish I had never worn...
I'm the first to admit I never had good taste when it came to clothes. I remember I was going to meet Alison's parents and put on a pair of bright yellow trousers which seemed to me quite smart and fashionable. When Alison arrived to pick me up she saw the trousers and a look of horror swept across her face. "You look like a canary," she said. On those rare occasions when I venture an opinion on matters of fashion in our family, Alison reminds me of those yellow trousers.

At the risk of being morbid, what song would you like played at your funeral?
I wouldn't want a song. For me it would have to be the W.H. Auden poem Funeral Blues which was used in the movie *Four Weddings and a Funeral.*

"The stars are not wanted now: put out every one;
Pack up the moon and dismantle the sun;
Pour away the ocean and sweep up the wood.
For nothing now can ever come to any good."

What was the low point of your career?
When Channel 7's *Today Tonight* program ran a story about laser surgery and defamed me. This was in 1998. I was very low that night. In fact the only person who rang me was my father who said "Really, it wasn't all that bad".

In their typical tabloid style, *Today Tonight* claimed we were taking risks without regard for the health and wellbeing of our patients. But what they said was simply wrong.

My partners – Chris Rogers and Gerard Sutton – and I took them to court and we won a resounding victory. One of the issues at that time was whether LASIK should be performed on both eyes on the same day, or whether they should be separated in time by a day, a week or a month. It was interesting seeing a clinical issue analysed by a Supreme Court

Judge, who very sensibly came down on the side of the information and the court ruled in our favour. We were just ahead of the curve. We understood the technology and knew that it was a very reasonable thing to perform surgery on both eyes on the same day; very convenient for patients, a much quicker recovery and just a sensible thing to do. Time has proven us right and within a few years, our protocol came to be considered the industry standard. The whole process was very character-building – a truly horrible thing to go through. It is the only time I've appeared in court, and indeed the only time I hope ever to do so.

If you weren't an ophthalmologist, what would be your dream job?
I always wanted to be a writer. I had dreams of being the next Ernest Hemingway, but it would have been disastrous. In my late teens / early twenties, when I was floundering and wondering what I was going to do with my life I wrote a number of short stories. They were dreadful.

If you were shipwrecked on a desert island, but you could take five books with you, which would they be and why?
Hemingway's *The Sun Also Rises*. I read that when I was twenty years old and loved it. I would take that because as a 'comfort' book, something beautiful from my youth which says so much by leaving unsaid all the seemingly important things. My second book would be Proust's *Remembrance of Things Past* because I may be on the island for a while and it will take ages to read. Also, it's something I always wanted to tackle, but have never had the time. Ulysses is my next choice. Although I've read it from cover to cover I didn't get it. Maybe the second time around something might click. My fourth choice would be *To Kill a Mockingbird* for the same reasons that I would take Hemingway.

My last book would be one that I read regularly. It's a strange book called *The Book of the Way* or *Tao Te Ching* written by Lao Tzu, a Chinese scholar in about 500 BC. It's a fabulous book of short verses beautifully written which talks about why the world is how it is and how to live your life. Even though it might seem a bit obvious in parts, given that it was written two and half thousand years ago makes it quite remarkable.

Which living person do you most admire?
Nelson Mandela, the captain of the ship that was his life.

As for someone who is personally known to me, our business partner, Dr Chris Rogers is someone for whom I have enormous respect and admiration. He has been one of the most important influences in my professional life. Together with Dr Peter Cohen, Chris and I brought the first excimer laser for short-sightedness to Australia in September 1991. His clinical knowledge is superb and his understanding of what mattered to patients helped us navigate our way through the early days of vision correction surgery in Australia. He was always willing to embrace new technology and take personal financial risks to do so if he thought it was in the best interests of his patients. Not many doctors, regardless of skill or experience have that pioneering spirit that drives them to constantly improve the way things are done, even at great personal cost.

I trusted Chris to perform LASIK on my own eye in 2005, and that has brought me fantastic freedom from reading glasses ever since. Chris's contribution to ophthalmology has been extraordinary. He has lived a very full and happy life with his wife and many children. An expert in thoroughbred horse racing and breeding, Chris also loves Russian literature and travel and is just one of those Renaissance men that society throws up from time to time. I am grateful to have been with him on this path.

How do you relax?
I relax by meditating, yoga and martial arts – all three. If I consciously have to relax for some reason, I will just quietly meditate for five to ten minutes before operating or before anything stressful.

Considering the huge advances with computers and mobile phones in the past thirty years, what do you think will be the most popular invention in 2050?
I think the thing that will become increasingly scarce will be personal privacy. By 2050 there will be some mechanism for regaining your privacy from the world so that the world you live in is not out there for everybody to see. This mechanism will retract your online life and most of us realise what fools we had made of ourselves in the previous thirty years.

If you were condemned to death by firing squad at dawn, but were allowed to choose your last meal, what would that be?
Nothing. I would face the firing squad having fasted for clarity of mind. I wouldn't want to miss what comes next.

> *I hear babies cry, I watch them grow,*
> *They'll learn much more than I'll ever know,*
> *And I think to myself, what a wonderful world.*

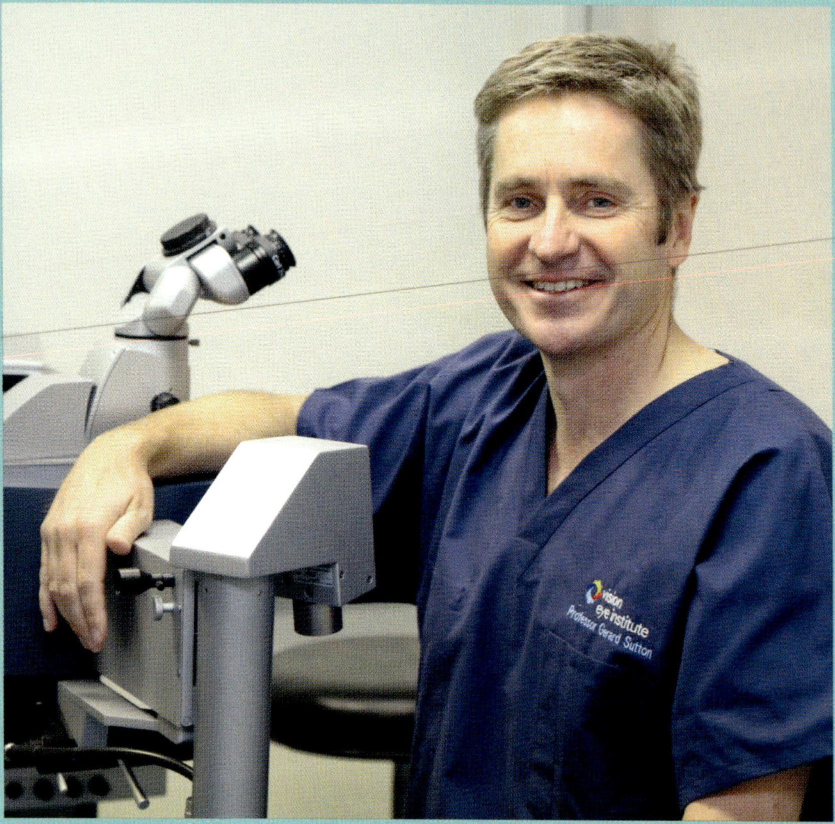
vision
eye institute
Professor Gerard Sutton

THE NAKED I
GERARD SUTTON

If you were condemned to death by firing squad at dawn, but were allowed to choose your last meal, what would that be?
My wife Gina's lamb roast washed down with a bottle of pinot noir from Central Otago, New Zealand. Most importantly it would be with my family and close friends.

Finish this sentence. "It's not fashionable to say this, but I love…"
Kiwis, Gough Whitlam and Tim Tams. New Zealanders have a carefree, stoic simplicity to them with a tough edge. I feel comfortable with them, share many of their passions for rugby, pinot noir and fly fishing and I enjoy their company. Gough had such great ideas and a brilliant sense of humour although execution in government was somewhat flawed. Tim Tams – no explanation required.

What is your earliest memory?
Our family lived in Lakemba, which was in those days a working class Irish Catholic neighbourhood. I remember we moved house when I was four years old. I had a thing for the girl next door and just as we were leaving I jumped out of the car and ran up and gave her a kiss. I never saw her again.

Is there a motto you live by?
No, but there are three principles I live by: to strive for excellence in everything I do, to suck the marrow out each day that life brings, and to help people along the way as best I can.

Which living person do you most admire?
My father. He managed to get the balance right in life. He has a great sense of humour, enjoys life but he has a social conscience and

contributed significantly to Australia in the field of education. Achieving that balance between enjoyment in life and vocational pursuits looks easy, but it isn't. I also have time for former President Bill Clinton. I felt that for all his failings he was generally trying to do the right thing for his people. I have yet to meet the perfect human being. I can identify with a flawed character like that but I strongly believe that everyone should get a chance at redemption.

Where is your favourite place in the all the world and why?
On the banks of the Tasman River running down from Mount Cook into Lake Pukaki on the South Island of New Zealand. On a sunny day with the snow-capped mountains in the background and trout in the river it is just the most stunning place. When I go fly fishing there I am able to forget about everything. Fly fishing is completely engrossing, so you have to concentrate on what you are doing. Sometimes, I'm just swept away by the natural beauty of the surroundings. It is a meditation of sorts. I lose myself in the grandeur and for once I can completely forget about work.

Fly fishing is completely engrossing, so you have to concentrate on what you are doing. Sometimes, I'm just swept away by the natural beauty of the surroundings. It is a meditation of sorts.

If they made a movie of your life who would be the best Hollywood actor to play you?
Harrison Ford. It was impossible not to love the character of Indiana Jones – this rugged, can-do college professor scouring the world in search of these priceless treasures, fighting tooth and nail to keep them out of the hands of the bad guys. If Harrison Ford was not available, my next choice would be Bradley Cooper – *The Hangover, Silver Linings Playbook, He's Just Not That Into You.* A few patients have told me I (*ahem*) look somewhat like him... although I don't see it myself.

Is there a person or a book or film or an event that changed your life?
There were many things that happened at various stages of my life which changed things for me. When I was a medical student I worked as a nurse's aide in a nursing home and that had a dramatic impact on my life. I was there for about six months and it certainly made me feel that I wanted to do something with my life that would alleviate suffering in some way.

Whenever I go to Burma my perception of what's important in life alters. It reinforces my desire to contribute in some small way. My first visit was to Cambodia in 1998 with Dr Geoff Cohn as part of a Fred Hollow's sponsored team. I saw the very best and the very worst of human nature. Altruism and self-sacrifice mixed with greed and sheer brutality. When we uncovered some unfortunate corruption amongst the hospital's administration we received death threats. The surgeons we helped train continue to perform sight-saving surgery.

Tell us something about you that very few people know.
I write poetry – not very well – but there you go. Only the threat of death would persuade me to quote even a single line here.

If you were shipwrecked on a desert island, but you could take five books with you, which would they be and why?
The first one I would take would be a fishing book – *How to Fish on a Desert Island* would be ideal, but I suspect there is no such book. However, Kevin Ireland's classic, *How to Catch a Fish* or Ernest Hemingway's *Old Man and the Sea* would be reasonable alternative. My next choice would be my favourite book, J.D. Salinger's *Catcher in the Rye*. I'd take that even though I probably know it off by heart. Third, *Lord of the Rings*, which was one of my favourites as a kid. From time to time I read it again. The fourth book would have to be something I could read again and again so it could only be a collection of Shakespearian sonnets. My last selection would be John Irving's *A Prayer for Owen Meany* which was given to me by a good friend and says just about all there is to say on growing up and dealing with one's fate.

What is your idea of perfect happiness?
I doubt that perfect happiness is achievable in this life. If it were, it would require a spiritual union with the universe in a mystical sense. The closest I come to this is either a certain stage of the evening at a barbecue with my family and friends or a solitary walk along a braided river on the South Island of New Zealand.

What do you consider the most overrated virtue and why?
The thing that springs to my mind is diplomacy, or to be more precise, people being unnecessarily diplomatic or over-cautious in their thoughts and opinions. For me frankness is a great virtue. I like people to say what they think and would much rather that than dealing with people who are insincere or guarded, leaving you with no idea what they really think.

What was the embarrassing thing that happened to you when you were growing up?
When it was discovered that I was learning ballet. At the time we were living in England and my two sisters were doing ballet. I had to hang around after school waiting for them so the teacher suggested I join in. I must admit I quite enjoyed hoofing around in my ballet gear until one day some mates turned up at the gymnasium after finishing footy training. Nothing much was said – It didn't need to be.

What is your most treasured possession?
My Sage 1 Ebony Black 7 weight fly fishing rod.

I wish I had never worn...
... leather pants. I was at a Year 11 party totally convinced I looked very groovy, but after a barrage of unflattering comments from males and females I never wore them again. In fact, they may not have even been real leather...

If you could invite five people from history to a barbecue at your place, who would they be and why?
I would like to have Mahatma Ghandi there because I believe he was one of the greatest figures of the 20th Century. Ghandi somehow combined the spiritual side of life with politics and then created a revolution by non-violent means. My second guest would be Ben Chifley. He is probably the closest we would ever come to in this country of having a Prime Minister who was genuinely a man of the people. His "The Light on the Hill" speech, which talks about working for the betterment of mankind, says it all. Third would be Harold Ridley, the pioneer of intraocular lens development. What a remarkable individual. He was highly regarded – then pilloried, ostracised, and condemned. Still he persisted with his ground breaking research and waited, not years, but decades for the recognition he deserved. Fourth, I would invite the French Impressionist painter, Auguste Renoir. I just love how he painted women. It seems to me that someone who can bring to life such famous party scenes as *Dance De La Galette* and *Luncheon of the Boating Party* would have to be a lot of fun to be with at party. And last of all I would have Louis Armstrong there playing his exquisite jazz which would make it a

> *I would have Louis Armstrong there playing his exquisite jazz, which would make it a barbecue to remember.*

barbecue to remember. Apart from liking jazz, the thought of him singing *What a Wonderful World* would be perfect. And I know that makes five, but I would like Bill Clinton to be there too to kick in with his saxophone and for entertainment value.

If you weren't an eye surgeon, what would be your dream job?
Professor of History at Sydney University.

What was the low point of your career?
There was a very near miss that could have been the low point of my career. Moorfields Eye Hospital in London, is regarded as THE place to train - certainly for Australian ophthalmologists. It is almost mythical in terms of its appeal having been set up after the Napoleonic wars to treat soldiers returning from overseas who had developed the eye disease called trachoma. One of my early career goals was to train at Moorfields. In 1996 I was working as a corneal fellow for Michael Lawless and Chris Rogers, which involved among many things, writing up papers for them. One of their cases was a patient whose medical history became hot property. He had had laser surgery (possibly not appropriately and not by Chris or Michael) and then had to have a corneal transplant. This involved removing a circle of tissue from his cornea and replacing it with a circle of tissue from a donor cornea. After the transplant was done we had this piece of the patient's cornea, which as it happened was one of the first pieces of tissue in the world that had undergone laser surgery which could be examined pathologically – hence being the medical equivalent of the Hope diamond. John Marshall, a professor in London who was the doyen of laser eye surgery, wanted that tissue and in the spirit of collegiality, Chris Rogers agreed to send it over. By coincidence I was travelling to the UK for an interview at Moorfields and offered to take the corneal tissue with me. Also, I calculated that it would give me a very good reason to meet Professor Marshall and maybe he might be grateful enough for the tissue to give me a job.

It just so happened that the Australian Ophthalmology Conference was in Kuala Lumpur that year. As I was invited to lecture there, I organised to stop in KL on my way to London. However, as it was one of the first ever lectures I had given, I was very nervous. Because this piece of corneal tissue was very precious and rare, I kept it with me all the time, even when I was giving the lecture. It all went really well and afterwards I felt this huge relief. The conference organisers arranged a tennis comp up in the mountains about an hour outside of KL. So after my lecture I went off to play tennis which was a lot of fun and I even managed to pick up a trophy.

We had this piece of the patient's cornea, which was one of the first pieces of human tissue in the world that had undergone laser surgery which could be examined pathologically – hence being the medical equivalent of the Hope Diamond.

We all had a few drinks and I was more than relaxed when I started getting ready to fly out to London that night.

Imagine how that calm, relaxed look on my face was abruptly shattered when I realised the corneal tissue was missing. I back-tracked my movements that day and realised I'd left it somewhere at the tennis courts up in the mountains. It was impossible for me to get back there and make my flight in time. My despair lifted when a pharmaceutical rep stepped in and offered to call the tennis club and try and locate the missing eye. Indeed they found the cornea sitting in its little sealed silver jar on the bar in the clubhouse. They put it in a taxi and it sent it to the airport. There seemed to be a million people checking in at KL airport that night and I couldn't imagine how the taxi driver was ever going to find me among this throng of people milling about the airport. By the time I'd checked in I'd given up all hope and kept imagining shaking hands with Professor Marshall and saying, "Corneal tissue? Sorry what corneal tissue was that?" Then over the PA I heard this announcement, "Dr Sutton please go to Gate 27." I looked down the concourse and there in the middle of the madding crowd was this little guy running in with a silver canister in his hand, just like an Olympic torch-bearer. "Over here," I bellowed, and in a swift exchange, I had the missing eye and he had a very large tip. Caught the flight to London, handed Professor Marshall the precious tissue and scored the job. Well honestly...

But theactuallowest point in my career occurred after I had passed all my exams to get into ophthalmology. I decided to take a few months off and hitch-hike around Europe. I arrogantly assumed that I would automatically be put onto the training program. Then when I was in Turkey I learned that I had not even been asked to do an interview. That was probably the lowest point for me. It was like my dream had been snatched away from me – that all that hard work had been for nothing. I remember thinking to myself that maybe ophthalmology was not for me and perhaps I should just bum around Europe for the next five years and enjoy myself. As it turned out there was some glitch in the system and I was then asked to go for an interview. Coincidentally, I learned that a young woman I really liked was going to be in Athens for forty-eight hours. I met up with her there and she is now my wife. In a way that period of time was the end of my youth and the beginning of a new part of my life.

What is your biggest regret?

One of my biggest regrets is that I didn't take my rugby more seriously. I always loved playing rugby and like a lot of schoolboys day-dreamed about playing for the Wallabies. After school I continued to play and while I briefly represented Norths under 21's in first grade I spoke to one of the coaching staff about my future in the game. He bluntly told me that I would never be big enough nor tough enough to play rugby at the top level. Reflecting on it now, his advice was probably correct, but I regret that I didn't pursue this dream anyway and find out for myself. That's why I always tell my children that they can achieve anything as long as they put the time and effort into it.

How do you relax?

Touch football and fishing. I play three or four times a week and although it's classified as a non-contact sport it can be a great outlet for any pent up frustration. I also like to have a cheap and cheerful dinner out with Gina and the kids at least once a week.

Finish this sentence. I'm very bad at....

...taking orders.

Tell us something about your co-author, Dr Lawless, that most people don't know.

Some doctors play golf, or tennis, but not Michael. He loves martial arts and when I first learned of this it seemed such a strange fit – that this quiet, thoughtful and certainly unaggressive man would be into karate. Michael told me he became interested in martial arts at university where he did what is known as 'full-contact' karate. Then, in his early forties he took up a different style of karate, Goju Ryu, and eventually obtained a black belt in this style. Michael says that his interest in karate was primarily in the way it works on the mind. When you 'fight' in karate time slows down and it's a very calm space in a sea of activity. It's exactly the space that you try and achieve when operating on an eye – you need clear thinking and to proceed exactly according to plan, but with a mind that's open to all possibilities that may occur.

At a martial arts event in 2010, Michael met an Aikido master and decided that this was a style he wanted to pursue. Aikido is a Japanese martial art, often called the "hippie" martial art because it relies on blending with an opponent and using their momentum, force and energy to defeat them. It has lots of joint locks for disabling opponents without killing them, which is why it's often used by Tokyo riots squads to subdue protestors. The aim is to convince an opponent that they no longer wish to resist you, it's futile. As Michael points out, this is sometimes very handy when dealing with partners in a group practice.

Michael has been one of the few Australian ophthalmologists who has achieved a genuine world-wide international reputation in refractive surgery. He is a meticulous surgeon and a great craftsman. In my opinion he is clearly one of the best refractive surgeons in Australia, if not the world.

At the risk of being morbid, what song would you like played at your funeral?
Throw Your Arms Around Me – Hunters and Collectors.

You will make me laugh and make me cry
And we will never forget it
You will make me call your name
And I'll shout it to the blue summer sky
And we may never meet again
So shed your skin and let's get started
And you will throw your arms around me
Yeah, you will throw your arms around me.

GLOSSARY

Artificial lens; (synonymous with **Intraocular lens**), an artificial lens implant, constructed of acrylic or similar material, implanted in the lens capsule of the eye during lens replacement surgery – either cataract or clear lens replacement.

Artificial tears; sterile eye drops used to lubricate the eye in the same way that natural tears do. They are used routinely after a vision correction procedure to lubricate the eyes to improve comfort as well as vision.

ASLA (Advanced Surface Laser); a form of vision correction surgery that reshapes the surface of the cornea using a cool, ultra-violet, excimer laser to correct long-sightedness, short-sightedness and astigmatism. Unlike LASIK, it does not involve the creation of a flap of corneal tissue, and is therefore the procedure of choice for thinner corneas. Although outcomes are equal to LASIK, recovery – both visual and comfort – is slower. It was formally known as PRK.

Astigmatism; a condition where the cornea is more highly curved in one contour that the other, resulting in a corneal shape more like a rugby ball rather than a regularly shaped soccer ball. This causes light entering the eye to be out of focus, resulting in blurred or ghosted vision.

Blended vision; the process by which one eye sees better for distance vision and the other for closer vision. It can occur naturally or can be accomplished with contact lenses or, increasingly, vision correction surgery.

Cataract; a loss of transparency or cloudiness of the natural lens within the eye that is caused most commonly by advancing age, as well as other factors such as exposure to UV light and certain medications.

Clear lens exchange; (synonymous with **Refractive lens exchange** and **Clear lens replacement**), a form of vision correction surgery where the clear contents of the eye's natural lens are removed and replaced with a smaller artificial lens of suitable power to correct for long- or short-sightedness, as well as astigmatism.

Clear lens replacement; (see **Clear lens exchange**)

Cornea; the clear, dome-shaped front surface of the eyeball that covers the iris and pupil. Due to its shape it bends light entering the eye so that it focuses on the retina at the back of the eye.

Corneal ectasia; the process of thinning and steepening of the central cornea after undergoing laser vision correction. Rarely seen these days, it is a potential complication of laser vision correction, particularly in the early days of the procedure, and one of the reasons why careful patient selection is so important.

Corneal inlay; a tiny device that is designed to be placed within the layers of the cornea in order to improve vision.

Crystalline lens; (see **Lens**)

Cryolathe; an instrument (now obsolete) designed by José Barraquer and used in early vision correction procedures. It was used to freeze microscopic sections of corneal tissue and then grind them to a new shape for clearer vision before replacing them in the patient's cornea.

Dominant eye; most people have a dominant eye, or one from which visual input is preferred. Even though you use both eyes to look at an object, your dominant eye is sending more information to your brain.

Endothelium; the inside layer of the cornea, which consists of a single layer of cells whose function is to regulate the cornea's hydration.

Enhancement procedure; a subsequent vision correction procedure carried out to reduce any residual error that may remain after an initial vision correction procedure is performed. It is typically required in 1–2% of cases.

Epithelium; the thin, outside layer of the cornea which protects the cornea. It is incredibly sensitive and grows rapidly, continually regenerating.

Excimer laser; a cool ultra-violet laser used in the LASIK and ASLA vision correction procedures to sculpt the cornea to the required shape to minimise dependence on spectacles. This laser delivers its energy in an extremely precise manner to vaporise tissue with virtually no generated heat or damage to the surrounding tissues.

Femtosecond; a unit of time equal to 10^{-15} seconds. It is the speed at which the femtosecond laser pulses energy to break the molecular bonds of the target tissue, thus separating it. It allows tissue to be cut without a blade ever touching the eye.

Flap (corneal); a microscopically-thin slice of corneal tissue that remains attached through a hinge of tissue. It is created with the femtosecond laser during the **LASIK** procedure and then folded out of the way so that the excimer laser can reshape the underlying cornea. It is then folded back into place where it adheres immediately without stitches. It allows the excimer laser to bypass the incredibly sensitive surface layer of the cornea.

Hyperopia; (see **Long-sightedness**)

Implantable lens; (synonymous with **Phakic intraocular lens**), an artificial lens implant which is implanted in the eye without the removal of the eye's natural lens. This does not disrupt the eye's ability (in the under 45s) to change its focus from distance to near and is a vision correction option for carefully selected younger patients who are not suitable for LASIK or ASLA.

Intraocular lens; (see **Artificial lens**)

IntraLase; the brand name for the first FDA (U.S.A.) approved femtosecond laser specifically used for the creation of the corneal flap in the first step in the **LASIK** procedure.

Iris; the coloured ring of muscular tissue that is behind the cornea and in front of the lens. It can dilate or constrict the pupil to control the amount of light entering the eye and is what gives the eye its characteristic colour.

Keratomileusis; any process of reshaping or sculpting the cornea. It can be mechanical reshaping, as in Barraquer's earlier procedures, or more recently, reshaping with the excimer laser as in the **LASIK** and **ASLA** procedures.

Laser cataract surgery; a form of cataract surgery where the cloudy contents of the eye's natural lens are removed and replaced with a smaller artificial lens to provide clear vision with minimum dependence on spectacles. This latest version of the cataract procedure uses a femtosecond laser to perform several steps of the procedure which were traditionally performed manually.

Laser lens surgery; a form of vision correction surgery where the clear contents of the eye's natural lens are removed and replaced with a smaller artificial lens of suitable power to correct for long- or short-sightedness, as well as astigmatism. Specifically, this procedure uses a femtosecond laser to perform several of the steps which were performed manually in previous lens replacement procedures.

LASEK; (not a term used in this book but, as it can cause confusion during research, it is included here), a term synonymous with **ASLA** and **PRK**.

LASIK; an acronym for laser in-situ keratomileusis, it is a form of vision correction surgery that involves the creation of a microscopically thin flap of corneal tissue that can be folded out of the way while a cool, ultra-violet, excimer laser reshapes the underlying corneal tissue to correct long-sightedness, short-sightedness and astigmatism. It has a very quick visual recovery and very little discomfort associated with it.

Lens; also called the **Crystalline lens** (and in this book, the natural lens), this is the transparent, jelly-like disc that sits behind your iris and is responsible for fine-tuning your focus from distance to near and everything in between. It becomes less flexible with increasing age and its ability to allow the eye to focus up close decreases progressively.

Long-sightedness; (or **Hyperopia**), this is a condition where either the cornea is too flat or the eyeball is too short so that light entering the eye is focused behind rather than on the retina. This results in near vision in particular being blurred.

Microkeratome; an oscillating metal blade previously used to create a very thin flap or slice of corneal tissue. Invented in the early days of vision correction surgery, it was used exclusively up until 2004 (in Australia) to create the flap in the first stage of the **LASIK** procedure. Since then it has been replaced with the IntraLase femtosecond laser which creates the flap without a blade ever touching the eye.

Micron; a measurement of length; there are a thousand microns in a millimetre.

Monovision; not a term used in this book but synonymous with **Blended vision**

Myopia; synonymous with **Short-sightedness** (or near-sightedness), this is a condition where either the cornea is too curved or the eyeball is too long so that light entering the eye is focused in front of rather than on the retina. This results in distance vision in particular being blurred.

Phakic intraocular lens; (synonymous with **Phakic IOL**, see **Implantable lens**)

Photo Refractive Keratectomy (PRK); a form of vision correction surgery (first performed in 1988) that reshapes the surface of the cornea using a cool ultra-violet, excimer laser to correct long-sightedness, short-sightedness and astigmatism. Unlike LASIK, it does not involve the creation of a flap of corneal tissue, and is therefore the procedure of choice for thinner corneas. Although outcomes are equal to LASIK, recovery – both visual and comfort – is slower. Modern **PRK** is called **ASLA** (Advanced Surface Laser).

Presbyopia; from the Greek words for 'elder sight', it is the deterioration of the ability to focus up close, which appears from middle age onwards and is caused by a loss in elasticity of the natural lens within the eye.

Pupil; the circular opening in the iris (the coloured part of your eye) through which light enters your eye. It is the 'black dot' you see in the middle of the iris.

Radial Keratotomy (RK); an obsolete form of vision correction surgery, begun in Russia and popular in the 1980's, in which the surgeon makes a series of thin cuts to the front surface of the cornea in a radial pattern – i.e. like the spokes of a bicycle wheel or the division of a pizza. The cuts, as they heal, cause the cornea to become flatter in the centre, thus correcting short-sightedness. It has been superseded by LASIK and ASLA.

Refractive error; the spectacle prescription needed to correct your vision.

Refractive lens exchange; not a term used in this book but synonymous with **Clear lens exchange** or **Clear lens replacement**. (See **Clear lens exchange**)

Refractive surgery; (see **Vision correction surgery**)

Residual error; any remaining short-sightedness, long-sightedness or astigmatism after a vision correction procedure has been performed.

Retina; the light-sensitive layer of cells which lines the inner back surface of the eye. It converts light reflected from the objects we see into electrical impulses, which are then sent along the optic nerves to the brain for interpretation. It can be thought of in a similar way to the film at the back of a camera.

Short-sightedness; (see **Myopia**)

SMILE laser; an acronym for small incision lenticule extraction, it is a form of vision correction surgery that uses a femtosecond laser to separate a thin, lens-shaped disc (or lenticule) of corneal tissue, which is then removed through a laser-created keyhole incision in the cornea. SMILE is used to correct moderate to high degrees of short-sightedness and astigmatism. It has a quick visual recovery and very little discomfort associated with it and it may be the procedure of choice for those with higher errors or drier eyes.

Stroma; the transparent collagen fibre layer which makes up over 90% of the cornea's thickness and provides the cornea with its structure and shape.

Tear film; a three-layer fluid film that coats the exposed surface of the open eye. It is vital to the health of the eye and functions to moisten, lubricate and protect the surface of the eye. Oxygen is also carried to the cornea through this film.

Vision correction surgery; synonymous with the term **Refractive surgery**, the umbrella term used to describe all forms of vision correction surgery, performed on a healthy eye with the goal of removing or reducing the need for glasses or contact lenses.

Visual acuity; a measurement of the sharpness or clarity of vision that enables us to resolve fine details.

APPENDIX

CLINICAL PAPERS BY THE AUTHORS

Eye & Vision 2015 April 2015, 2:7

Intraocular lens power calculation following laser refractive surgery

Hodge C, McAlinden C, Chan C, **Lawless M**, **Sutton G**, Martin A

ABSTRACT

Refractive outcomes following cataract surgery in patients that have previously undergone laser refractive surgery have traditionally been underwhelming. This is related to several key issues including the preoperative assessment and intraocular lens power calculations. Peer-reviewed literature is overwhelmed by the influx of methodology to manipulate the corneal or intraocular lens (IOL) powers following refractive surgery. This would suggest that the optimal derivative formula has yet been introduced. This review discusses the problems facing surgeons approaching IOL calculations in these post-refractive laser patients, the existing formulae and programs to address these concerns. Prior published outcomes will be reviewed.

By 1997 Drs Lawless and Sutton were amongst the first to publish their data recognising the effect of laser refractive surgery on intraocular lens calculations. Almost 20 years later ophthalmology has made tremendous progress however concerns still remain. In this review article, Dr Lawless and Dr Sutton have been asked to share their wealth of experience with general ophthalmology in tackling this potentially difficult issue.

J Cataract Refract Surg. 2015 Mar;41(3):683-6.

Incidence of cystoid macular edema: femtosecond laser-assisted cataract surgery versus manual cataract surgery.

Levitz L, Reich J, Roberts TV, **Lawless M.**

ABSTRACT

In recent years cataract surgery has undergone significant change with the introduction of laser-assisted procedures. The risks and benefits of this technology have previously been explored and published by Dr Lawless and colleagues. This recent study represents the largest analysis of a potential vision-threatening postoperative complication and serves as a well-measured source for ophthalmic surgeons considering the uptake of this technology.

Clin Experiment Ophthalmol. 2014 Nov;42(8):796-8.

Investigation of keratoconus in an Australian refractive population.

Hodge C, Chan C, **Sutton G.**

ABSTRACT

Unfortunately not all patients represent excellent candidates for laser refractive surgery. Keratoconus is a corneal eye disease which represents a strict contraindication to laser surgery. In this paper Dr Sutton reviewed his significant database of patients seeking refractive surgery to determine the relative incidence of patients found to have this complex disease and thereby be counselled against surgery. This represents a first for the Australian population with the results suggesting that the disease may be more common than previously indicated internationally.

Int Ophthalmol Clin. 2013 Winter;53(1):111–28. doi: 10.1097/IIO.0b013e31827134 6e.

LASIK.

Lawless M, Hodge C.

SYNOPSIS

Approximately 25% of the world's population (with up to 70% in some Asian countries) will require some form of vision correction for distance activities. LASIK surgery represents a significant alternative for many of this population. Since the initial laser vision correction procedures were performed in 1983, refractive surgery has undergone significant developments. This article reviews the many changes across time and describes the respective clinical outcomes in dealing with these refractive errors. Recent meta-analyses suggests that the overall satisfaction rate for LASIK is 96% which reflects the excellent results now obtained.

International Ophthalmology Clinics is a quarterly journal that publishes subject-specific issues on topics of immediate interest to ophthalmologists worldwide. Publication in the journal is by invitation only and represents acknowledgement of leadership in the particular field.

Ophthalmology. 2013 Feb;120(2):227–33. doi: 10.1016/j.ophtha.2012.10.026. Epub 2012 Dec 6.

Surgical outcomes and safety of femtosecond laser cataract surgery: a prospective study of 1500 consecutive cases.

Roberts TV, **Lawless M**, Bali SJ, Hodge C, **Sutton G.**

ABSTRACT

Objective: To report the surgical outcomes and safety of femtosecond (FS) laser cataract surgery (LCS) with greater surgeon experience, modified techniques, and improved technology.

Participants: Fifteen hundred consecutive eyes undergoing FS laser cataract and refractive lens exchange surgery in a single group private practice.

Methods: All eyes undergoing LCS between April 2011 and March 2012 were included in the study. Cases underwent anterior capsulotomy, lens fragmentation, and corneal incisions with the Alcon/LenSx FS laser (Alcon/LenSx, Aliso Viejo, CA). The procedure was completed by phacoemulsification and insertion of an intraocular lens. The cases were divided into 2 groups: Group 1, initial experience consisting of the first 200 cases; and group 2, the subsequent 1300 cases performed by the same surgeons.

Results: Both groups were comparable for baseline demographic parameters. Anterior capsule tears occurred in 4% and 0.31% of eyes, posterior capsule tears in 3.5% and 0.31% of eyes, and posterior lens dislocation in 2% and 0% of eyes in groups 1 group 2, respectively ($P<0.001$ for all comparisons). Number of docking attempts per case (1.5 vs 1.05), incidence of post-laser pupillary constriction (9.5% vs 1.23%), and anterior capsular tags (10.5% vs 1.61%) were significantly lower in group 2 ($P<0.001$ for all comparisons).

Conclusions: In the authors' experience, the surgical outcomes and safety of LCS improved significantly with greater surgeon experience, development of modified techniques, and improved technology.

SYNOPSIS

Femtosecond laser cataract surgery has been one of the most significant advances within ophthalmology in recent history. Vision Eye Institute received the 3rd laser unit in the world in April 2011 and since then Drs Lawless and Sutton have lectured widely, both internationally and at home, on the early experience and results.

Ophthalmology is rated the most prestigious journal in peer-reviewed ophthalmology. This article represents a landmark paper that suggests, for the first time, that laser cataract surgery is indeed as safe as, and in many cases significantly safer than manual surgery techniques.

Curr Opin Ophthalmol. 2013 Jan;24(1):3–8. doi: 10.1097/ICU.0b013e32835a936b.

Femtosecond cataract surgery: transitioning to laser cataract.

Sutton G, Bali SJ, Hodge C.

ABSTRACT

Purpose Of Review: The introduction of the femtosecond laser to the field of cataract surgery offers many potential benefits. The femtosecond laser is able to perform three important steps in cataract surgery: capsulotomy, lens fragmentation and corneal incisions. Although evidence in support of its efficacy is accumulating, there is a surgical learning curve that needs to be addressed. This review outlines key issues to consider when contemplating the transition to laser cataract surgery in clinical practice.

Recent Findings: Laser cataract surgery has been shown to be associated with an initial learning curve. Femtosecond lasers produce a more accurate and precise anterior capsulotomy, improve intraocular lens centration and reduce intraocular lens tilt. Visual and refractive outcomes, although in a limited number of studies, have been shown to be at least as good as those of conventional phacoemulsification. The impact of reduced phacoemulsification energy on the corneal endothelium is still being investigated.

Summary: The automation of key steps by the use of femtosecond lasers in cataract surgery has several potential advantages. Emerging literature supports the transition from conventional phacoemulsification to the laser cataract surgery.

SYNOPSIS

Peer-reviewed literature remains the essential forum for specialists to gain an unbiased understanding of current concepts. *Current Opinion in Ophthalmology* is an international journal that discusses the latest surgical techniques and technology. Authorship of articles is by invitation only and inclusion suggests that the authors themselves stand at the forefront of the topic.

Here Dr Sutton discusses the promising recent introduction of femtosecond laser to cataract surgery and its capacity to improve on the standard manual technique.

Ophthalmology. 2012 May;119(5):891–9. doi: 10.1016/j.ophtha.2011.12.025. Epub 2012 Feb 22.

Early experience with the femtosecond laser for cataract surgery.

Bali SJ, Hodge C, **Lawless M**, Roberts TV, **Sutton G.**

ABSTRACT

Objective: To describe the intraoperative complications and to evaluate the learning curve with femtosecond laser cataract surgery.

Methods: The initial 200 eyes undergoing cataract surgery between April 2011 and June 2011 by 6 surgeons were included in the study. The cases underwent anterior capsulotomy, lens fragmentation, and corneal incisions with the femtosecond laser. The procedure was completed by phacoemulsification and insertion of an intraocular lens. Data were collected about patient demographics, preoperative investigations and intraoperative complications. The cases were divided into 4 groups–group 1 included the first 50 cases, group 2 included cases 51 through 100, group 3 included cases 101 through 150, and group 4 included cases 151 through 200–and were analyzed.

Results: The mean age of patients included was 69.2±9.8 years. Of the 200 eyes, 74.5% underwent a complete procedure of laser capsulotomy, lens fragmentation, and corneal incisions. Five eyes had suction breaks during the laser procedure that led to the remainder of the laser procedure being aborted. Twenty-one (10.5%) eyes showed the presence of small anterior capsular tags. The number of eyes with free-floating capsulotomies was 35 (17.5%). The other complications during the study were anterior radial tears (n = 8; 4%), posterior capsular ruptures (n = 7; 3.5%), and dropped nucleus (n = 4; 2%). A significant difference was noted among the sequential groups with respect to the number of docking attempts ($P<0.001$), miosis after the laser procedure ($P<0.001$), and free-floating capsulotomies ($P<0.001$), suggesting an improving learning curve. The surgeons with prior experience with femtosecond lasers had fewer complications in the first 100 cases ($P<0.001$). No difference in complications was observed after the initial 100 cases.

Conclusions: In this case series, there was a clear learning curve associated with the use of femtosecond lasers for cataract surgery. Adjustment to surgical technique and prior experience with a femtosecond laser seemed to flatten the learning curve.

SYNOPSIS

The introduction of new technology is not without the potential for issues or complications. By describing the learning curve, and offering possible solutions, the doctors at Vision Eye Institute were able to provide vital information for all surgeons within ophthalmology.

J Cataract Refract Surg. 2011 Oct;37(10):1884–94. doi: 10.1016/j.jcrs.2011.05.029.

Photorefractive keratectomy with mitomycin-C after corneal transplantation for keratoconus.

Hodge C, **Sutton G, Lawless M**, Rogers C.

ABSTRACT

Purpose: To evaluate the efficacy of photorefractive keratectomy (PRK) for residual refractive error after penetrating keratoplasty (PKP) for keratoconus.

Method: Consecutive patients who had PRK augmented with topical mitomycin-C (MMC) after PKP for keratoconus were retrospectively reviewed. Patients were divided into a a low cylinder group (refractive cylinder ≤ 6.00 D) and a high cylinder group (refractive cylinder >6.00 D). Visual acuity, refraction, and keratometry were analyzed preoperatively and 1, 3, 6, and 12 months postoperatively.

Results: The study comprised 47 eyes (41 patients). The spherical equivalent (SE) decreased from -4.24 D ± 3.23 (SD) preoperatively to -0.71 ± 1.03 D 12 months postoperatively in the low cylinder group and from -4.19 ± 3.54 D to -2.45 ± 3.42 D, respectively, in the high cylinder group. The refractive cylinder decreased from -4.27 ± 1.4 D to -1.71 ± 1.55 D, respectively, in the low cylinder group and from -7.78 ± 1.21 D to -4.6 ± 2.54 D, respectively, in the high cylinder group. By the last follow-up, 8.3% of patients had lost 2 lines of corrected distance visual acuity. There were no cases of corneal haze greater than 2+ or of graft rejection.

Conclusions: Penetrating keratoplasty with adjunctive MMC decreased several refractive variables in patients with previous PKP. These results compare well with those in the published literature and suggest PRK is as effective as, and probably safer than, laser in situ keratomileusis in treating refractive error in these cases.

SYNOPSIS

Evaluating surgical techniques remain central to the development of better outcomes. The treatment of patients following previous surgery remains difficult with those patients at particular risk of related complications. LASIK remains the popular choice for surgeons and patients and accounts for approximately 90% of all laser refractive procedures. Surface ablation or PRK represents the initial procedure developed by surgeons. Here we have shown that despite surface ablation representing an earlier technique, in combination with recent laser technology, it appears to represent potentially a more accurate and safer option for these patients. Understanding the subtle differences in techniques allowed the surgeons to assess and describe these changes for the wider ophthalmic community.

Curr Opin Ophthalmol. 2011 Jul;22(4):238–44. doi: 10.1097/ICU.0b013e3283477c9c.

Applications of the femtosecond laser in corneal refractive surgery.

Kim P, **Sutton GL**, Rootman DS.

ABSTRACT

Purpose Of Review: The femtosecond laser has become a rapidly and widely adopted technology for surgeons performing refractive surgery. With the advances in femtosecond lasers, clinical outcomes and safety with their use have improved. The purpose of this review is to outline the current surgical applications of the femtosecond laser in corneal refractive surgery.

Recent Findings: Many surgeons have adopted femtosecond technology for the creation of the laser in-situ keratomileusis flap secondary to its improved safety, precision and reproducibility. Other applications include astigmatic keratotomy, channel creation for the insertion of intrastromal corneal ring segments, femtosecond lenticule extraction, facilitating the insertion of corneal inlays as well as in intrastromal presbyopia correction (IntraCOR). Further novel applications continue to be developed.

Summary: This review outlines the recent advances and applications of the femtosecond laser in corneal refractive surgery.

SYNOPSIS

Laser technology has developed at a significant pace over recent years and now provides many options for surgeons treating a range of patients. Here Dr Sutton and co-authors were asked to update ophthalmologists throughout the world on this rising technology. This article in particular foreshadowed the major development and impact of femtosecond laser technology in cataract surgery.

J Cataract Refract Surg. 2011 Mar;37(3):603–7. doi: 10.1016/j.jcrs.2010.12.036.

Keratectasia following LASIK in a patient with uncomplicated PRK in the fellow eye.

Hodge C, **Lawless M, Sutton G.**

ABSTRACT

We present a case of unilateral keratectasia in a laser refractive surgery patient. Laser in situ keratomileusis (LASIK) was performed in the first eye, but because of difficulty lifting the femtosecond-created cap in the second eye, photorefractive keratectomy was performed in that eye. Neither eye had risk factors for keratectasia; both had identical low scores on the Randleman risk factor score. Although femtosecond laser caps were created in both eyes, ectasia developed in only the LASIK eye, in which the cap was lifted. We believe this is the first case of this complication reported in the literature. It highlights our incomplete knowledge of the risk factors for keratectasia following LASIK and suggests that unlifted flaps do not undergo the same biomechanical weakening as flaps that are lifted.

SYNOPSIS

Complications, although infrequent, may still occur despite taking recommended precautions. Recognizing particularly unusual cases represents a significant opportunity to teach the wider community about these rare cases and is essential to increasing our understanding. This case recognized a world first and assisted the confirmation and development of a software program designed to assist surgeons screen for at-risk patients.

(Retrospective testing of a new method for detecting ectasia-susceptible corneas. Saad A, Hodge C, Lawless M, Gatinel D. J Cataract Refract Surg. 2011 Oct;37(10):1907-8)

Clin Experiment Ophthalmol. 2010 May;38(4):335–40.

External analysis of the Randleman Ectasia Risk Factor Score System: a review of 36 cases of post LASIK ectasia.

Chan CC, Hodge C, **Sutton G.**

ABSTRACT

Background: To validate Randleman's model of ectasia risk factor scores using a large unbiased sample of unpublished cases.

Methods: Data were collected retrospectively on 36 eyes with ectasia post laser in situ keratomileusis treated by two surgeons at Vision Eye Institute. The data were then entered into Randleman's risk factor score system. Data were also collected about posterior maximum elevation (PME) and posterior maximum elevation position (PMEP); and these were compared with a control group of 50 eyes.

Results: Of the 36 eyes, 9 (25%) were classified as low risk, 7 (19%) as moderate risk and 20 (56%) as high risk. On average, the most points were scored in the topography and topography was abnormal in 69% of cases. Topography points also correlated the most strongly with the increasing risk scores ($P < 0.0001$).PME or PMEP was not significantly different between our ectasia group and the control group.

Conclusion: Randleman's ectasia risk factor scale can miss a significant proportion of patients at risk of ectasia. Other factors must play a role in ectasia risk. Abnormal corneal topography appears to be the most important preoperative risk factor.

SYNOPSIS

Ectasia represents a significant potential complication following laser surgery that may dramatically affect visual acuity. As such the possible risk factors for this condition have been heavily investigated. In this paper we reviewed an existing ectasia score system and suggest an enhancement to the system. These findings have been replicated by other authors since.

J Refract Surg. 2008 Oct;24(8):802–6.

Accuracy and precision of LASIK flap thickness using the IntraLase femtosecond laser in 1000 consecutive cases.

Sutton G, Hodge C.

ABSTRACT

Purpose: To report the safety and flap thickness predictability of LASIK using the IntraLase femtosecond laser.

Method: A retrospective analysis of 1000 consecutive LASIK cases was performed to assess the rate of intra- and postoperative complications and loss of best spectacle-corrected visual acuity (BSCVA). A subset of 260 eyes was prospectively analyzed to assess flap thickness predictability using subtraction ultrasound on the day of surgery.

Results: No serious intra- or postoperative complications were noted. Three (0.3%) patients had epithelial defects that required a bandage contact lens. Four (0.4%) patients had slipped caps on day 1 that required repositioning. Two (0.2%) patients developed grade I diffuse lamellar keratitis. No patient developed epithelial ingrowth >1 mm from the flap edge, transient light sensitivity, or infection. No patient lost > or = 2 lines of BSCVA at 6 months postoperatively. With an attempted flap thickness of 105 microm with the 15-KHz laser, the mean flap thickness was 116.79 +/- 10.75 microm (range: 95 to 148 microm) (n = 119). In the 30-KHz group (n = 141), the target corneal flap thickness was 115 microm, with a mean flap thickness of 114.02 +/- 9.82 microm (range: 93 to 163 microm). Overall 87.3% of eyes were within +/- 20 microm of the intended result. Ninety-eight percent of caps created with the 30-KHz laser were within +/- 20 microm compared to 74.8% in the 15-KHz group.

Conclusions: LASIK surgery with the IntraLase femtosecond laser is safe and flap thickness is predictable.

SYNOPSIS

Continual review is important to assess the validity of various technologies. Here Dr Sutton observed the safety and predictability of creating the LASIK flap by femtosecond laser in a large sample of patients. This confirmed the superiority of this technology against previous methods. The paper has been referenced numerous (>30) times in the peer-reviewed literature as a result.

J Refract Surg. 2006 Nov;22(9):S965–8.

Fulfilling the promise of laser refractive surgery.

Lawless MA, Potvin RJ.

ABSTRACT

Purpose: To review the characteristics required to perform accurate and precise laser refractive surgery relative to the current state of the art and the technology improvements needed in the future.

Method: The general characteristics for laser refractive surgery are identified and their relative contributions to a successful result considered. For each characteristic, the degree to which improvements in technology are likely to improve results is discussed.

Results: The environment (surgeon, site), technology (laser, aberrometer), and patient are identified as key factors affecting results. Although aberrometers appear to be clinically sufficient, improvements in laser beam characteristics and delivery should improve system consistency. Current registration technology may be a factor in variability from patient to patient, but the greatest contribution in this regard would appear to be patient biomechanical and healing response factors.

Conclusions: Wavefront-guided laser refractive surgery has demonstrated an ability to be better than conventional surgery. Improvements in laser technology, registration technology, and biomechanical diagnostics are expected to further improve results. These potential improvements are expected to reduce variability and suggest that the final potential of this technology has not yet been realized.

SYNOPSIS

Understanding the application of any technology is essential to its use with patients. This paper provided an excellent summary for the international ophthalmic audience regarding wavefront-guided laser surgery. Wavefront or customized surgery suggests that the surgeon is able to optimize the treatment for the patient's individual aberrations and refractive error. This has had a significant impact on outcomes and continues to evolve to present day. Dr Lawless has been intimately involved with these developments over time.

J Cataract Refract Surg. 2005 May;31(5):979–86.

Laser in situ keratomileusis for refractive error after cataract surgery.

Kim P, Briganti EM, **Sutton GL**, **Lawless MA,** Rogers CM, Hodge C.

ABSTRACT

Purpose: To evaluate the safety and efficacy of laser in situ keratomileusis (LASIK) to correct refractive error following cataract surgery.

Methods: This retrospective study reviewed 23 eyes (19 patients; 10 female, 9 male) treated with LASIK for refractive error following cataract surgery. The Summit Apex Plus and Ladarvision excimer laser and the SKBM microkeratome were used. The mean age was 63.5 years (range 50 to 88 years). The mean length of follow-up was 8.4 months (range 1 to 12 months) and mean interval between cataract surgery and LASIK was 12 months (range 2.5 to 46 months).

Results: The mean preoperative spherical equivalent refraction (SEQ) for myopic eyes was -3.08 +/- 0.84 diopters (D) (range -4.75 to -2.00 D) and for hyperopic eyes was +1.82 +/- 1.03 D (range +0.75 to +3.00 D). The mean improvement following LASIK surgery was greater for myopic than hyperopic eyes (myopic, 2.54 +/- 1.03 D versus hyperopic, 1.73 +/- 0.62 D; P=.033). The percentage of patients within +/-0.5 D of intended refraction post-LASIK surgery was 83.3% for myopic eyes and 90.9% for hyperopic eyes and all eyes were within +/-1.0 D of intended (P<.001). The percentage of eyes with uncorrected visual acuity of 20/40 or better in the myopic group improved from none preoperatively to 91.7% postoperatively (P<.001) and in the hyperopic group improved from 27.3% preoperatively to 90.9% postoperatively (P=.008). No eyes lost 2 or more lines of best corrected visual acuity.

Conclusion: Laser in situ keratomileusis appears to be effective in correcting refractive error following cataract surgery. Longer-term studies are required to determine refractive stability.

SYNOPSIS

Cataract surgery has developed significantly over the past 20 years. Numerous developments in technology, techniques and lens calculations have provided surgeons with excellent results that are starting to rival laser refractive surgery for success. A small minority of patients will not achieve the desired refractive or visual end point. For some of these patients laser surgery may provide an opportunity to further reduce or remove the dependence on optical aids following surgery. This paper explored the results in hyperopic or long-sighted patients following cataract surgery and confirmed that these patients can expect excellent results following the enhancement procedure.

J Refract Surg. 2004 Jan–Feb;20(1):10–9.

Development of a questionnaire to assess subjective vision score in myopes seeking refractive surgery.

Fraenkel G, Comaish IF, **Lawless MA**, Kelly MR, Dunn SM, Byth K, Webber SK, **Sutton GL**, Rogers CM.

ABSTRACT

Purpose: To assess vision in patients with myopia and myopic astigmatism before and after refractive surgery.

Methods: A prospective controlled study of visual quality amongst myopes and astigmatic myopes. Focus groups, ophthalmic surgeons, and questionnaire experts devised a Subjective Vision Questionnaire (SVQ), modified after a pilot trial. Participants were administered the SVQ before clinical evaluation. Items answered by over 95%, with factor loadings > 0.55 were included. Test-retest reliability was assessed by repeat testing. Factor analysis identified groups of questions measuring particular dimensions of data.

Results: Sixty-seven items were answered by 128 patients and reduced to 24 items in a final questionnaire. Factor analysis identified six types of questions within the questionnaire, the most important of which was related to driving.

Conclusion: The simplicity, low cost, and psychometric properties of the Subjective Vision Questionnaire support its use clinically and in research.

SYNOPSIS

The quality of a patient's vision following refractive surgery can often be overlooked by an examiner. The existence of complications such as haloes or glare may significantly reduce the overall satisfaction of a patient despite an excellent refractive result. Here we designed a questionnaire to assess the subjective outcome in patients undergoing laser surgery. The questionnaire remains relevant today and is used both in our practice and around the world to help surgeons quantify what the patient sees in real-world terms.

J Refract Surg. 2003 Nov–Dec;19(6):S691–6.

Laser in situ keratomileusis with Alcon CustomCornea.

Lawless MA, Hodge C, Rogers CM, **Sutton GL**.

ABSTRACT

Purpose: To report the 3-month results of our first cases of laser in situ keratomileusis (LASIK) with Alcon's CustomCornea.

Methods: Wavefront analysis was performed using the LADARWave aberrometer and ablation was performed with the LADARVision4000 system. Thirty-one eyes of 17 patients were analyzed prospectively, at 1 and 3 months after CustomCornea surgery. Psychophysical tests were performed, including high and low contrast acuity, and contrast sensitivity under scotopic and photopic conditions. In addition, psychometric testing was performed using a subjective vision questionnaire.

Results: Mean spherical equivalent refraction improved from a baseline -3.05 +/- 1.92 D to +0.02 +/- 0.28 D at 3 months (28 eyes). At 3 months, 46.4% (13 eyes) had uncorrected visual acuity of 20/16, 92.7% (26 eyes) had 20/20, and 100% (28 eyes) had 20/25 uncorrected visual acuity. Three months after CustomCornea surgery, there was a statistically significant improvement in contrast sensitivity under both scotopic and photopic conditions, and a statistically significant increase in third and fourth order aberrations. There was a statistically significant improvement in visual quality as measured by the subjective vision index, increasing from a preoperative mean 66.62 to 87.63 at 3 months after surgery.

Conclusions: CustomCornea was an improvement over conventional LASIK as measured by most psychophysical and psychometric parameters. The relationship between higher order aberrations and other psychophysical and psychometric measurements needs more analysis.

SYNOPSIS

As discussed previously, customized laser technology has provided a number of potential advantages for the surgeon and patient over previous techniques. This paper represented the first time in world, peer-reviewed ophthalmic literature that customized laser ablations provided tangible benefits over standard laser technology.

Br J Ophthalmol. 2002 Jul;86(7):815–22.

The surgical correction of moderate hypermetropia: the management controversy.

McGhee CN, Ormonde S, Kohnen T, **Lawless M**, Brahma A, Comaish I.

SYNOPSIS

This review in the highly respected British Journal of Ophthalmology investigated the opinions of several surgeons regarding current laser technology for patients who were long-sighted. The opening introduction confirmed Dr Lawless' standing amongst his peers.

"Four experienced ophthalmic surgeons who have undertaken cornea and refractive fellowships and have a combined experience of more than 10,000 refractive surgical procedures were asked to consider the best options for this hypothetical subject."

J Cataract Refract Surg. 2002 May;28(5):775–81.

Laser in situ keratomileusis for residual myopia after photorefractive keratectomy.

Comaish IF, Domniz YY, **Lawless MA**, Webber SK, Rogers CM, **Sutton GL**.

ABSTRACT

Purpose: To evaluate the efficacy and safety of laser in situ keratomileusis (LASIK) for myopic regression and undercorrection after photorefractive keratectomy (PRK).

Methods: Fifty eyes of 32 patients were treated by LASIK for residual myopia following primary PRK. The mean spherical equivalent refraction (SEQ) was -2.92 diopters (D) +/- 1.57 (SD) (range -0.75 to -7.88 D). The mean refractive cylinder was 0.96 +/- 0.74 D (range 0 to 3.50 D). For analysis, the eyes were divided into 2 groups: those with 0 or low corneal haze (Group 1) and those with severe corneal haze (Group 2). In Group 1, the SEQ was -1.99 +/- 0.79 D (range -0.75 to -3.75 D) and in Group 2, -3.77 +/- 1.62 D (range -0.75 to -7.90 D). The procedure was performed using the Chiron Automated Corneal Shaper and the Summit Apex Plus laser. The mean interval between PRK and LASIK was 25 months (range 9 to 59 months). The following parameters were studied before and after LASIK retreatment: SEQ, mean refractive cylinder, uncorrected visual acuity (UCVA), and best corrected visual acuity (BCVA). Complications after LASIK retreatment were evaluated.

Results: Six months after LASIK, the mean SEQ in all eyes was -0.65 +/- 0.86 D (range +1.50 to -3.35 D); 70.0% of eyes were within +/-1.00 D of emmetropia and the UCVA was 6/12 or better in 72.5%. The mean SEQ in Group 1 was -0.22 +/- 0.55 D (range -0.88 to -1.50 D) and in Group 2, -0.97+/- 0.92 D (range 0.12 to -3.25 D); the UCVA was 6/12 or better in 94.0% of eyes in Group 1 and in 56.0% in Group 2. No statistically significant between-group difference was found in lines of Snellen acuity lost or gained at 6 months. No eye lost more than 1 line of BCVA.

Conclusions: Laser in situ keratomileusis appears to be a safe, effective, and predictable procedure for treating eyes with 0 or low haze with residual myopia after PRK. It is less predictable in eyes with severe haze.

SYNOPSIS

The treatment of residual error is not always straight forward with a number of factors requiring investigation and analysis. This paper reviewed a number of patients who had previous surface ablation or PRK that required retreatment procedures to obtain improved unaided outcomes. In this series the surgeons completed LASIK over the initial ablation with excellent results albeit in patients without significant prior complications. Understanding the most appropriate approach remains central to effective outcomes.

Curr Opin Ophthalmol. 2002 Feb;13(1):7–13.

Phakic intraocular lenses.

Comaish IF, **Lawless MA.**

ABSTRACT

Since Zaldivar's review of phakic intraocular lenses in these pages in 2000, further reports of experience with this technology have emerged. Their relative advantages and disadvantages over competing technologies are becoming clearer. Clinical trials, including Food & Drug Administration (FDA) trials, have shown predictability, stability, and efficacy. Safety of these implants over the long term remains a concern, but in some situations, at least, phakic intraocular lenses are becoming the refractive correction of choice. This brief review looks at the most recent data to emerge regarding phakic intraocular lenses.

SYNOPSIS

Phakic IOLs have been around for some time in various formats. These lenses are inserted either in front or directly behind the iris of the eye and coexist with the natural lens of the eye. Commonly these lenses remain most appropriate for patients with large refractive errors or those who may not be suitable for laser technology. Here Dr Lawless was asked to review the current advantages and disadvantages of the lenses and provide an overview of an emerging technology which is still utilized today.

J Refract Surg. 2001 Sep–Oct;17(5):505–10.

Recutting the cornea versus lifting the flap: comparison of two enhancement techniques following laser in situ keratomileusis.

Domniz Y, Comaish IF, **Lawless MA**, Rogers CM, **Sutton GL**.

ABSTRACT

Purpose: To evaluate enhancement techniques following laser in situ keratomileusis (LASIK).

Methods: Recutting was performed on 263 eyes and the flap was lifted in 55 eyes that had LASIK for simple myopia or myopic astigmatism. The time interval between LASIK and retreatment was 340+/-46 days (range, 270 to 892 days) in the recutting group and 215+/-36 days (range, 53 to 617 days) in the flap lifting group. Mean spherical equivalent refraction, refractive cylinder, uncorrected and best spectacle-corrected visual acuity were examined prior to, and 1, 3, and 6 months after retreatment.

Results: Seventeen eyes were lost to follow-up in the lifting group and 53 eyes in the recutting group. In the recutting group, mean spherical equivalent refraction improved from -1.48+/-1.25 D to -0.49+/-0.88 D at 6 months. In the flap lifting group, mean spherical equivalent refraction improved from -1.05+/-1.49 D to -0.45+/-0.39 D at 6 months. Refractive cylinder did not change significantly in either group (P = .2). There was a significant increase in uncorrected visual acuity (UCVA) of 6/6 in each group. In the recutting group, UCVA of 6/6 increased from 3.8% to 65.2% at 6 months, and in the lifting group from 3.6% to 71.1% at 6 months. In the recutting group, seven free flaps and three macerated flaps that required removal occurred. One eye in the recutting group and two in the lifting group developed significant epithelial ingrowth. No patient lost more than one line of best spectacle-corrected visual acuity (BSCVA).

Conclusion: Both procedures were safe, effective, and highly predictable for enhancements, but flap complications may be more likely with recutting.

SYNOPSIS

Inevitably a small number of patients will be left with a residual error following surgery. As previously stated, understanding the most appropriate and safest methods for treating these errors is paramount to obtaining excellent final outcomes. This paper investigated two different techniques for treating patients requiring an enhancement procedure. Although both techniques appeared effective in refractive terms; re-lifting the previous flap suggested an overall safer method. This technique remains the standard today for surgeons throughout the world.

Br J Ophthalmol. 1999 Sep;83(9):1013–8.

LASIK for post penetrating keratoplasty astigmatism and myopia.

Webber SK, **Lawless MA, Sutton GL**, Rogers CM.

ABSTRACT

Aims: To report the results of a series of patients who were treated with LASIK to correct post penetrating keratoplasty ametropia.

Methods: 26 eyes of 24 patients underwent LASIK to correct astigmatism and myopia after corneal transplantation; 14 eyes also received arcuate cuts in the stromal bed at the time of surgery. The mean preoperative spherical equivalent was -5.20D and the mean preoperative astigmatism was 8.67D.

Results: The results of 25 eyes are reported. The mean 1 month values for spherical equivalent and astigmatism were -0.24D and 2.48D respectively. 18 eyes have been followed up for 6 months or more. The final follow up results for these eyes are -1.91D and 2.92D for spherical equivalent and astigmatism. The patients undergoing arcuate cuts were less myopic but had greater astigmatism than those not. The patients receiving arcuate cuts had a greater target induced astigmatism, surgically induced astigmatism, and astigmatism correction index than those eyes that did not. One eye suffered a surgical complication. No eyes lost more than one line of BSCVA and all eyes gained between 0 and 6 lines UCVA.

Conclusions: LASIK after penetrating keratoplasty is a relatively safe and effective procedure. It reduces both the spherical error and the cylindrical component of the ametropia. Correction of high astigmatism may be augmented by performing arcuate cuts in the stromal bed.

SYNOPSIS

Patient demand for improved vision has continually driven the surgical techniques and technology. This paper highlights the continued improvement in the treatment of patients with significant refractive error following corneal transplantation. The doctors at Vision Eye Institute incorporated a further surgical step for these patients to augment the effects of the laser. This became widely used within ophthalmology until further advances in technology were available.

J Refract Surg. 1997 Jul–Aug;13(4):362–6.

Intraocular lens power calculation for cataract surgery after photorefractive keratectomy for high myopia.

Kalski RS, Danjoux JP, Fraenkel GE, **Lawless MA**, Rogers C.

ABSTRACT

Objective: To assess intraocular lens (IOL) power calculations in patients undergoing cataract surgery after excimer laser photorefractive keratectomy (PRK) for myopia.

Methods: Four eyes of two patients underwent phacoemulsification with IOL implantation after PRK for myopia. The estimated refractive error that would have been induced had the IOL predicted for emmetropia been implanted was calculated using SRK-II, SRK/T, Holladay, and Binkhorst formulas. Manual keratometry and videokeratography-simulated keratometry values measured before surgery were used. Keratometry values calculated by subtracting the refractive change induced by the excimer laser PRK from the manual keratometry or videokeratography-simulated keratometry values measured before PRK were also used. Both spectacle and corneal plane calculations were performed.

Results: Manual keratometry and videokeratography-simulated keratometry values underpredicted the IOL power. Corneal plane manual or videokeratography refraction-derived keratometry calculations were most accurate using the SRK/T formula, while spectacle plane calculations were most accurate using the SRK-II formula. In both methods the calculated refractive error was within 0.52 diopters (D) for the emmetropic lens power predicted. Statistical analysis was not performed.

Conclusions: Refraction-derived keratometric values provided the most accuracy in calculating IOL powers. Our results suggest the SRK/T formula was the most accurate for corneal plane calculations, while the SRK-II formula was the most accurate for spectacle plane calculations.

SYNOPSIS

It wasn't too long before the initial patients undergoing laser surgery required cataract surgery. The curvature of the cornea is a significant factor in calculating the power of the lens to be inserted in the eye following cataract removal. As this had been dramatically altered with laser surgery there was a significant impact upon early cataract results.

This paper was one of the first to recognize the effect of laser on the calculations for cataract surgery, particularly in patients with previously high myopia. Understanding this issue was paramount to obtaining better results following cataract surgery.

J Refract Surg. 1996 Jan–Feb;12(1):61–7.

Comparison of 5-mm and 6-mm ablation zones in photorefractive keratectomy for myopia.

Kalski RS, **Sutton G**, Bin Y, **Lawless MA**, Rogers C.

ABSTRACT

Background: Variation in ablation zone diameter may alter visual acuity and/or refractive effect in photorefractive keratectomy. Despite theoretical benefits of using a smaller diameter ablation zone, clinical studies suggest that a larger ablation zone may decrease problems associated with photorefractive keratectomy.

Methods: The results of our initial 34 consecutive eyes treated with a 5-mm diameter ablation zone using a Summit Technology ExciMed UV200LA excimer laser were compared retrospectively to our initial 34 consecutive eyes treated with a 6-mm diameter ablation zone using a Summit OmniMed excimer laser. Eyes had a spherical equivalent refraction between -1.00 and -6.00 diopters (D) and astigmatism less than 1.00 D. Patients were followed for a minimum of 6 months.

Results: Eyes treated with a 6-mm ablation zone had less hyperopia and a spherical equivalent refraction closer to emmetropia at 1, 2, and 3 months ($P = 0.001$). Eyes treated with a 6-mm ablation zone had better uncorrected visual acuity at 1 and 2 months ($P = 0.001$). Less subepithelial haze was noted at 2 months ($P = 0.01$) and 3 months ($P = 0.002$) in the 6-mm group. At 6 months postoperatively, 30 of 32 eyes (94%) treated with a 6-mm ablation zone had a spherical equivalent refraction within 0.50 D of emmetropia, and all 32 eyes (100%) were within 1.00 D of emmetropia; in the 5-mm ablation zone group, 28 of 34 eyes (80%) were within 0.50 D and 29 (85%) were within 1.00 D of emmetropia. Patients treated with a 6-mm ablation zone complained less of night halos and had fewer differences between night and day vision.

Conclusions: In this study of myopia of -1.00 D to -6.00 D, eyes treated with a 6-mm ablation zone achieve a more rapid visual recovery with less variation in refractive outcome and less adverse effects than those treated with a 5-mm ablation zone.

SYNOPSIS

Early lasers were limited in how they may ablate the eye. Small diameter laser beams could potentially leave a patient with significant haloes and glare under night or dim conditions. The impact upon the healing process was also unknown at this time.

This paper was significant to the progression of our understanding the effect of laser beam profiles. Soon after this paper was published, laser surgeons worldwide transitioned to the larger ablation zones with better refractive and patient quality results.

Aust N Z J Ophthalmol. 1994 Nov;22(4):243–7.

Refractive keratoplasty for post-graft astigmatism.

Whitehouse G, **Sutton G, Lawless MA**, Rogers C.

ABSTRACT

Refractive keratoplasty using modified relaxing incisions with compression sutures was performed on 33 patients with high post-keratoplasty astigmatism. The mean reduction in keratometric astigmatism was 8.38 dioptres from a preoperative mean of 12.21 dioptres (SD, 3.59) to 3.93 dioptres (SD, 2.13). All patients noted a marked functional improvement. Two patients required reoperation. One patient required resuturing. Our modification of undercutting the relaxing incisions greatly increases the range of astigmatism that can be treated with this technique.

SYNOPSIS

As surgeons became familiar with laser technology the boundaries were rapidly extended. For patients who had corneal transplantation for eye disease, large residual refractive errors were routine following surgery. As glasses often remained unable to fully correct these errors, the patient was often left with poor vision.

Although these results suggest that patients were still left with a small error following laser surgery, this was then correctable with glasses or contact lenses providing clarity of vision not initially possible.

J Refract Corneal Surg. 1994 Mar–Apr;10(2 Suppl):S171–3.

Photorefractive keratectomy for myopia of more than -10 diopters.

Rogers CM, **Lawless MA**, Cohen PR.

ABSTRACT

Twenty-seven consecutive eyes of 18 patients with myopia of more than -10.00 diopters (D) were treated by photorefractive keratectomy (PRK) using the ExciMed UV200LA excimer laser and a double ablation technique in an attempt to achieve a refraction of plano. The preoperative mean spherical equivalent refraction was -13.32 D (standard deviation 2.54, range -10.25 to -20.50). Preoperative spectacle corrected visual acuity ranged from 6/6 to 6/60 and one eye had had two previous refractive keratotomies. Follow up ranged from 3 to 15 months (mean 8.9). At 6 months after surgery, the mean change in refraction was 11.03 D, from a preoperative mean of -13.32 D to a postoperative mean of -2.29 D. The mean keratometric flattening was 5.83 D, from a preoperative mean of 42.92 D to a postoperative mean of 39.09 D. The reason for this large difference is uncertain. At three months the mean spherical equivalent refraction was +0.07 D (SD 2.94, range -10.50 to +3.25). The 14 eyes that had achieved 12 months follow up had a mean spherical equivalent of -1.91 D (SD 3.87, range -11.00 to +2.50). Seven of these 14 eyes have been reablated for manifest scars in association with regression. All 14 eyes had best spectacle corrected visual acuity at or better than their preoperative level.

SYNOPSIS

Technology advanced relatively quickly expanding the potential range of treatment. A prescription of -10 diopters represents extreme myopia. These results suggested that laser surgery could dramatically reduce the dependence on optical aids for such patients providing a significant difference for such patients' quality of life.

Refractive options for patients with extreme myopia have been superseded by further technology however this study highlighted an important step in surgeons understanding of the treatment in these cases.

Med J Aust. 1993 Oct 18;159 (8):535, 538.

Excimer laser photorefractive keratectomy: 12 months' follow-up.

Lawless MA, Rogers C, Cohen P.

ABSTRACT

Objective: To report the results of 12 months' follow-up of patients with myopia treated with excimer laser photorefractive keratectomy.

Design: A prospective study of patients undergoing excimer laser photorefractive keratectomy for myopia was commenced in September 1991. The study included 50 eyes (38 patients) with preoperative myopia of -1.50 to -6.00 dioptres and a maximum astigmatism of 0.75 dioptres.

Results: Forty-six (92%) of the 50 eyes had an uncorrected acuity of 6/6 or better at 12 months, and 49 eyes (98%) had 6/12 or better. No patients had lost their best corrected acuity at 12 months. Forty-five eyes (90%) were within 0.50 dioptres of emmetropia and 47 eyes (94%) were within 1.00 dioptre of emmetropia.

Conclusions: Excimer laser photorefractive keratectomy is a safe and predictable procedure for low to moderate myopia. It will increasingly be offered to patients as an alternative to the use of spectacles and contact lenses.

SYNOPSIS

This study represents the data from the original cases of refractive laser in Australia. Although the technology would be classified as basic in current times, the results provide excellent results albeit in a limited sample.

This is the starting point for the refractive laser industry in Australia. The doctors at Vision Eye Institute were at the forefront of technology in the early 1990s and remain so now.

REFERENCES

1.
The Lancet, Vol 379, Issue 9827, 5–11 May 2012, pages 1739–1748
Myopia
Prof Ian G Morgan, Prof Kyoko Ohno-Matsu MD, Prof Seang-Mei Saw PhD

2.
American Journal of Epidemiology, 1980 May; Vol 113, Issue 1, pages 62–80
Racial variations in vision
Hugh R Taylor

3.
Evolutionary Anthropology 9 (4): 156–185. (2000)
A theory of Human Life History Evolution: Diet, Intelligence and Longevity
Hillard Kaplan, Kim Hill, Jane Lancaster, and A. Magdalena Hurtado

4.
Journal of Cataract and Refractive Surgery. 2013 Jul; 39 (7): 1047–58
Laser in situ keratomileusis in United States Naval aviators.
Tanzer DJ, Brunstetter T, Zeber R, et al
Navy Refractive Surgery Center, Naval Medical Center, San Diego, California, USA

5.
Ophthalmology 2008 Oct; 115(10):1655–62
The Incidence of Contact Lens–Related Microbial Keratitis in Australia
Fiona Stapleton, PhD, Lisa Keay, PhD, Katie Edwards, BAppSc (Optom), et al
Institute for Eye Research, Sydney, Australia.

ACKNOWLEDGEMENTS

M.L

First, I must thank Audrey Molloy, who kept bringing us all back to our readers' needs rather than our own, and managed in that effortless way of hers to 'translate' scientific jargon into what I hope is readable and enjoyable prose. Likewise Graeme Brosnan, a friend for many years and an expert editor. At the beginning of this project I think I surprised him when I pointed out that ultimately our friendship was more important than any book, and that whatever happened along the journey, nothing was to harm our friendship. I feel like I have won on all counts because it was a pleasure to work together on this book and we remain good friends.

Also, of immeasurable value to me were my first real 'teachers': Professor Doug Coster in Adelaide, Professor Richard Troutman in New York, and of course the late Professor José Barraquer in Bogota. They were incredibly generous with their time and gave me professional advice, which has helped me throughout my career. Mention must also be made of Professor Dick Lindstrom in Minneapolis who encouraged me to get involved with the International Society of Refractive Surgery, and Professor Frank Martin, a source of sage advice so many times over the years.

Another to whom I am deeply indebted is Dr Chris Rogers, my professional partner in this journey of refractive surgery. He was and remains a perfect foil to my personality and together we have been able to achieve much more than we could have as individuals. Chris has always been there when I needed him, whether to give his unique perspective, or simply to make me appreciate the humour of many situations in which we found ourselves. A special thanks to Matt Metcalfe who was with me from the beginning of the laser cataract journey in Budapest.

I would also like to thank all my fellow speakers at so many meetings and conferences around the globe; you are my ophthalmic international family. Many like Michael Knorz and Zoltan Nagy, have become real friends, and they have been a profound influence on my career as well as my understanding of medicine. Credit must also go to my Karate Master Kenshu Watanabe, and my Aikido Master Bruce Robertson. They provided me with the focus and balance to help me live a life and to be a better surgeon. Many a time I have arrived at Aikido training feeling a bit tense and irritable and they have shown me how to shut out all the unimportant things and concentrate on the things that matter.

All my partners and staff at Vision Eye Institute Chatswood and Bondi Junction deserve special thanks, including Phillip Lu , Nancy Tsang, Shih Shih Ta, Megan Freeman, Des Kom, Layla Moshrif, Cecilia Wei, Rosie Kim, Jane Nolan and many others. Thank you Dr Tim Roberts and Dr Jeff Friedrich, my partners at Chatswood from almost the beginning, and a special thanks to Dr Colin Chan for having the courage to join us so early in his career. Also, it would be remiss of me not to thank Anne Hänseler for working tirelessly, interpreting and typing my work over two decades. We are a team that works well together and I am eternally grateful for all your help. Liz Feeney, my anaesthetist for many years and Jo-Ann Dean, who runs the best operating room, bar none, deserve special thanks, as does Catherine Sulman for working alongside me and being unfailingly cheerful.

I thank the Board of Vision Eye Institute for allowing me to practice in the way that I do, and I thank Cathie Searle, our manager at Chatswood for tolerating me. They have been a great support to me and my colleagues. Another I must thank is Chris Hodge our Director of Research. He is so methodical, intelligent and understated, always preferring to shun the limelight, but Chris always delivers.

More important than anyone or anything I must thank my wife Alison and our three children Anna, Harry and Will. Obviously I'm biased, but I happen to think they are the greatest. I doubt I could have done it without the wisdom, patience, humour and forbearance of Alison. My family has tolerated my physical absences over the years, as well as my preoccupation with work even when at home. They have made it all worthwhile.

Finally, I would like to salute my colleague and co-author, Gerard, who I greatly admire for his skills as a surgeon as well as for being unfailingly enthusiastic from the very beginning of this project.

Dr Michael Lawless

ACKNOWLEDGEMENTS

G.S

Many people have worked very hard to put this modest book together. I would firstly like to thank Audrey Molloy, without whose dedication and hard work this book would not have been possible. As well as contributing many of the ideas, Audrey was like a breath of fresh air and I believe her good humour somehow made its way onto the pages of this book. She is a true friend. I would also like to extend my thanks to Graeme, our editor, who has consistently steered this book along the right course and ultimately, if it is found to be readable, digestible and, God forbid, entertaining, then Graeme and Audrey will be responsible for that.

Thank you to our Director of Research Chris Hodge, our typist Anne Hänseler and my personal assistant Kati Kenny, all of whom gave unselfishly of their time and expertise. It is fair to say that Kati has organised my working life over the last three years and anything I have managed to achieve has in no small way been as a result of her organisational skills. Thank you to the wonderful staff and doctors at Vision Eye Institute Chatswood, my colleagues and my friends, who help provide our patients with an unparalleled level of ophthalmic service. Thanks also to my optometric and ophthalmic colleagues who have trusted me with their patients' care and who share the challenges and the triumphs in helping them see.

I would also like to thank those of my mentors who shared their surgical knowledge with me over the years. In particular, I would like to thank Professor Frank Martin, Professor John Marshall, Professor Gottfried Naumann, Dr Jeff Friedrich, Dr Pauline Rumma and Dr Justin Playfair. Thanks to Professor Geoff Crawford and Professor Graham Barrett in Perth, Professor Doug Coster in Adelaide, Associate Professor Colin Chan at our practice in Sydney, and to Professor Charles McGhee and Professor Helen Danesh-Meyer at Auckland University who provided academic and life support at times when none was forthcoming on this side of the ditch. These surgical professors taught me that the best eye surgeons are those that are not afraid to question the status quo, who make medical decisions based on facts and who above all else pursue surgical excellence.

I would also like to thank the Dean of Medicine at Sydney University, Professor Bruce Robinson, and Dr John Gregory-Roberts who have supported this type of surgical professorial work through the Sydney Medical School Foundation Chair of Corneal & Refractive Surgery at Sydney University.

Thank you to Dr Geoff Cohn, my mentor in developing-world ophthalmology, who, together with Sister Barbara Roberts, has shared with me and guided me through what, at times, seemed like the insurmountable challenges of practising ophthalmic surgery in Cambodia and Burma. Also, I would like to thank my co-author, Michael, for being there when it mattered. He will always be my benchmark in surgical expertise.

I would also like to thank my friends and fly fishing mentors Brian Butler, Henare Dewes, Will Spry, John Gilmore, Gordon Sanderson and Rick Arnheim who have introduced me to the mystical rivers of the South Island of New Zealand and shared their vast knowledge with me.

Special mention must be made of my parents Gerard and Sylvia for their guidance and example that service and vocation enrich lives. I consider myself most fortunate to have grown up in the wonderful family environment they created.

To my wife and best friend Gina, my children Katie, Ben and Rosie, I extend my deepest thanks, for tolerating my absences, my occasional distance and my shortcomings as a husband and a father. You are never far from my thoughts and your love provides the inspiration for everything I do.

If you are one of the people who helped bring this book to life, and I have somehow neglected to mention you, please accept my apologies for that oversight. But it is a fact that many, many people helped in ways they may not have realised – by making an astute comment on a draft – or by offering an opinion on the illustrations – or by simply offering support when decisions had to be made. You know who you are, so once again thank you all.

Finally, thank you to my patients, for the honour and privilege of looking after you and being able to share in the joy of your new vision.

Prof Gerard Sutton

DR MICHAEL LAWLESS MBBS, FRANZCO, FRACS

Michael Lawless is recognised worldwide as an authority in laser eye surgery. He specialises in laser vision correction, laser cataract and corneal transplant surgery. Michael has performed over 25,000 surgical procedures and has always combined a busy surgical practice with clinical research and innovation.

In 2014 Dr Lawless and his colleagues at Vision Eye Institute were the first in Sydney to perform the new SMILE laser procedure. It was also in 2014 that Dr Lawless was asked to join the invitation-only American Ophthalmological Society. The AOS is arguably the world's most prestigious club for ophthalmologists who have contributed to the science and practice of ophthalmology through their careers. Dr Lawless' thesis for the AOS will involve a study of cataract and intraocular lens surgery to identify the best methods of improving intraocular lens power selection.

In 2013, in combination with Alcon/LenSx, Michael was the focus for the "operating room of the future"; an attempt to bring a level of precision and refinement to laser cataract surgery under one roof as a show-case for the Asia Pacific region. Over a period of several months, Michael will be involved in teaching the region's best ophthalmologists as they make a steady stream to the Vision Eye Institute surgery in Chatswood, Sydney.

Background

The son of a builder, Michael went to Marist Brothers at Lidcombe and Auburn and completed his schooling at St Joseph's College, Hunters Hill. "From the time I was a small boy in primary school I wanted to be a doctor. The doctor in our community in Sefton in the western suburbs of Sydney was someone who was respected and intelligent and seemed to do good work. I just wanted to be like that. It was my good fortune that I knew what I wanted to do with my life. It is the easiest thing in the world once you work out what you want to do, because all you have to do is work towards that goal."

Michael attended the University of Sydney where he graduated in Medicine in 1980. After completing his residency at Royal Newcastle Hospital, Michael joined the Royal Australian Navy. He did officer training at HMAS Creswell and was then posted to *HMAS Cerberus*. When he was successful with his entrance exams for ophthalmology, the navy agreed to release him as they were keen to retain his future services as a consultant ophthalmologist. When he became an ophthalmologist Michael served on the Ophthalmology Consultative Committee for the combined Australian Defence Forces, a role he continues with to this day.

After completing ophthalmology training in Sydney, Michael did two years of sub-specialty education – a Corneal and External Diseases Fellowship with Professor Doug Coster in Adelaide and a second Fellowship in Corneal and Refractive Surgery with Professor Richard Troutman at the Manhattan Eye, Ear & Throat Hospital in New York. He also travelled to Colombia to work with the legendary Dr José Barraquer. In 1988 Michael left New York and returned to Sydney and set up practice as a corneal transplant surgeon. Then, in 1991, together with Dr Chris Rogers and Dr Peter Cohen, he brought the first excimer laser into Australia.

Professional Credentials

His career highlights include:

- First Australian surgeon to perform laser cataract surgery with the femtosecond laser in February 2011
- Performed the first LASIK procedure in Sydney in 1995
- President, International Society of Refractive Surgery, 2001

- Chairman, Department of Ophthalmology, Royal North Shore Hospital and Northern Area Health Service, 2000-2006
- Over 100 publications in the peer reviewed scientific literature and textbook chapters written on innovations in eye surgery
- Selected to perform televised live surgery at international meetings, including the American Academy of Ophthalmology, the American Society of Cataract and Refractive Surgery and the Asia Pacific Academy of Ophthalmology
- 2006 – 2014, Medical Director, Vision Eye Institute
- 2014 to present, Clinical Associate Professor, University of Sydney Medical School.

His many awards include:

- Cedric Cohen Medal for Excellence in the Royal Australian College of Ophthalmologists examination, 1982
- Visiting Professor, University of Melbourne, 1998
- Founders Award from the International Society of Refractive Surgery, Chicago 2005
- Senior Honour Award, American Academy of Ophthalmology for Services to Education in Ophthalmic Surgery, 2012
- Dr Lawless is frequently invited to be a Guest Lecturer at the world's main scientific meetings. He is also consultant ophthalmologist to the Australian Defence Force and consultant ophthalmologist to the NSW Rugby Union.
- In 2016 Dr Lawless has been invited to be the guest speaker at both the All Indian Ophthalmological Society and the Indonesian Ophthalmological Society.

Beyond Work

Michael is married with three children and is a Shodan (black belt) in Goju Ryu karate. He currently trains in Aikido and practices yoga. He has also taken on an active role in educating ophthalmologists through the American Academy and the Asia Pacific Academy of Ophthalmology. He coordinates their cataract educational programs for the Asia/Pacific area including China and India. ●

PROFESSOR GERARD SUTTON MBBS, MD (AUCK), FRANZCO

Gerard Sutton is the Inaugural Professor of Corneal and Refractive Surgery at Sydney University. His appointment to the Chair in 2009 was a reflection of his international reputation as a surgical expert in laser vision correction, laser cataract and corneal transplant surgery.

Gerard is first and foremost an ophthalmic surgeon. To date, he has successfully performed around 20,000 surgeries. His chief strength is as an innovator who critically analyses new technologies in order to provide the best and safest surgical options for his patients.

Background

Born in Lakemba, Sydney, Gerard's father was an engineer in the Royal Australian Navy who went on to become Vice Chancellor of Wollongong University. During Gerard's boyhood years, the family spent several years in England and the United States. Whilst in school, Gerard considered entering the priesthood. However, that notion vanished when puberty struck. He then narrowed down his career options to going into medicine or playing rugby for Australia – preferably both at the same time. He was to achieve only one of these goals. In 1993 Gerard completed his ophthalmic training at the Sydney Eye Hospital, where he is now Professor of Corneal and Refractive Surgery. In 1996 he completed advanced surgical training at St Thomas' and Moorfields Eye Hospital in London and The Friedrich-Alexander University in Erlangen, Germany, having received the DAAD and RANZCO Sigma scholarships. Gerard thus became the first Australian to complete overseas fellowship training in laser refractive surgery.

Professional Credentials

His career highlights include:

- Gerard is the Sydney Medical School Foundation Professor of Corneal and Refractive Surgery at the Save Sight Institute, University of Sydney
- He is currently the Medical Director of The Lions NSW Eyebank
- He is a consultant to the Royal Australian Navy
- Visiting Professor, University of Medicine, Mandalay

His previous appointments include:

- Inaugural Corneal and Refractive Fellow at Vision Eye Institute Chatswood in 1994
- Chief Ophthalmologist for the Sydney 2000 Olympics
- Chief surgeon in NSW for the Artificial Cornea project in 2002
- Member of the Australian Council of Healthcare Standards for LASIK in 2002–2005

Gerard has introduced many new surgical techniques to Australia, as well as achieving many milestones in his career. They include:

- First Australian surgeon to complete overseas fellowship training in laser eye surgery
- First surgeon in Australia to perform LASIK using the IntraLase femtosecond laser
- First surgeon in Australia to use Intracorneal Ring Segments for the treatment of keratoconus
- First Australian surgeon to perform a corneal transplantation using the femtosecond laser
- First Professor of Corneal and Refractive Surgery in Australia
- Established the first remote university degree in refractive surgery in the world
- First Australian appointed to the Council of Asia Cornea Society

- Fellow of Academy of Asia-Pacific Professors of Ophthalmology (1 of only 50) 2015
- Asia Pacific Academy of Ophthalmology Achievement Award 2015
- Over 100 peer-reviewed papers and textbook chapters
- First surgeon (with his colleagues) to perform SMILE laser procedure in Sydney

Gerard has published over 80 peer-reviewed papers and textbook chapters, and continues to lecture both nationally and internationally. He was a Visiting Professor to the Victorian Eye and Ear Hospital in 2007, and in 2009 was Visiting Professor at The Eye Institute, Auckland and Visiting Professor (1st Australian) University of Medicine Mandalay 2015. He has also been a Visiting Professor to Otago University since 2010. He has given many keynote and invited lectures internationally in recent years including: World Cornea Congress San Diego 2015, World Ophthalmology Conference Mexico 2016, World Ophthalmology Conference Tokyo 2014, Asia Society of Cataract and Refractive Surgery Singapore 2013, American Academy of Ophthalmology Chicago 2012, and Asia Pacific Academy of Ophthalmology Busan 2011.

Beyond Work

Gerard lives with his wife Gina, his three children Katie, Ben and Rosie and a dog called Charlie. He is a keen fly fisherman and touch footballer.

Gerard has worked overseas in a volunteer capacity on numerous occasions. In Cambodia he helped train doctors in cataract surgery, which was the major cause of blindness in that part of the world. On one occasion he was asked to take some corneas to Burma to teach a particular type of corneal transplant. When he arrived at the monastery hospital in Wachet, there were thousands of people queued up and all he had was five corneas. Five would have their sight restored – the rest would remain blind. This sobering experience reinforced Gerard's realisation that as one person he could make a difference, not by flying in for a brief stay to perform surgery but by teaching local surgeons how to do the surgery themselves.

There is an old Chinese proverb which rings true for him on many levels: "Give a man a fish and you feed him for a day. Teach a man to fish and you feed him for a lifetime". Gerard returns to Burma regularly to teach corneal and cataract surgery in Mandalay. ●